INTERMITTENT

FASTING FOR WOMEN

New Healthier Eating Habits That Will Detox Your Body, And
Reset Your Metabolism To Lose Weight

by SUSAN AVEDON

Table of Contents

Introduction

Intermittent Fasting has been on the rise in popularity, and more scientific studies are being done to explore the benefits of it. It is basically cycling between eating periods and fasting periods. This will cover how Intermittent Fasting can help women with weight loss. The benefits are endless! Intermittent Fasting can help with:

- **Weight loss:** Intermittent Fasting is a great strategy for weight management. Many people find that once they begin Intermittent Fasting, they naturally eat less because they aren't hungry and don't have cravings for unhealthy foods. This is because Intermittent Fasting lowers insulin and leptin levels, along with other metabolic signaling pathways in the body. These changes cause a dramatic decrease in appetite and make you feel much fuller than those who are following normal diets but are feeling hungry all the time. We have found that women are more likely to lose weight when they adopt Intermittent Fasting.

- **Diabetes:** the biggest concern for people with diabetes is keeping stable glucose levels, preventing damage to their blood vessels. By reducing insulin levels as well as leptin levels, Intermittent Fasting is beneficial for women who are dealing with diabetes. It has also been shown to protect women from heart disease and stroke as well.

- **Regular menstrual cycles:** many women still struggle with having a regular cycle even while taking birth control pills or other forms of hormone treatments due to health problems or other reasons. Intermittent Fasting may help many women restore normal menstruation by regulating hormone production.

There are many other reasons to do intermittent fasting. Whether you are fighting disease, weight loss, or just want to feel better, I hope you take a look at Intermittent Fasting as a method to help you with whatever you are going through.

The different approaches to Intermittent Fasting involve a cycle of eating and fasting. The number of cycles, the duration of each fast, and the interval between cycles can vary depending on the approach. One approach is to eat for 10-12 hours each day and fast for about 14-16 hours. Another is to restrict food intake on alternate days (i.e., every other day).

The Alternate-Day Diet involves restricting food intake on alternate days (i.e., every other day). For example, a woman might follow the pattern of eating 500 calories a day for five days, followed by a fast day of not eating. The next day, she might eat all she wants until she has eaten as much as she can comfortably fit in her stomach and then go into fasting mode where she does not eat anything for two to three hours. This pattern would repeat itself periodically during the week until the woman reaches her goal weight.

The Anti-Inflammatory Diet involves eating specific foods over four days, followed by a four-day fast. On day 1, the "fasting" diet includes vegetables such as arugula, broccoli, kale, and spinach. Fish like sardines can be included too. On days 2 and 3 of the "fasting" diet, more vegetables are allowed, along with other foods that include ginger root and turmeric powder. For example, a vegetarian might have rice with cottage cheese for one meal and bread with vegan turkey slices for another meal. On day 4 of the "fasting" diet, you get to eat any food you want until you are satisfied.

The Fast Mimicking Diet is a protocol that involves consuming a special liquid diet for five days each month, while fasting for two days in between. It was pioneered by Dr. Valter Longo of the University of Southern California, and has been shown in preliminary studies to reduce metabolic and oxidative damage related to aging, as well as symptoms of several metabolic and autoimmune diseases.

The Fasting Mimicking Diet is another form of intermittent fasting that involves consuming only black coffee or water during the day, with three meals eaten at night. In studies on mice it has been shown to delay age-related declines in cognition and prevent some types of cancer.

I am often asked about Intermittent Fasting for women. Before I answer this question, let's first take a look at what doctors think about it. Studies found that Intermittent Fasting might be beneficial for people with type 2 diabetes, and it can help the participants lose weight. Another study found that this eating pattern may lower insulin levels and lead to weight loss in obese individuals who have high cholesterol levels.

The effects of Intermittent Fasting on other metabolic parameters, such as blood pressure, triglycerides, or glucose tolerance, were less clear from those studies. More studies are needed to assess whether the potential health benefits of Intermittent Fasting in normal weight or overweight adults outweigh any potential negative effects.

When it comes to answering the question of whether Intermittent Fasting for women is safe, there are mixed answers. Some studies found that a short period of fasting, such as 16 hours, may not be dangerous for people with metabolic syndrome. Other studies didn't find any negative effect of short-term fasting on blood pressure or insulin resistance in healthy adults.

On the other hand, long-term fasting may increase the risk of obesity and diabetes in people with risk factors such as insulin resistance and abdominal fat stores. Fasting may also cause problems if it is repeated every day or less frequently. If it is repeated every other day, the body adapts to the rhythm in a supportive way. It may prevent too much weight loss and cause hunger. Those studies found that people who fasted more than 23 days a month increased their risk of type 2 diabetes.

Most physicians, however, believe that Intermittent Fasting can be beneficial for people who have health issues related to a high-calorie diet or those who are trying to lose weight. The effects of Intermittent

Fasting on blood pressure, cholesterol levels, or glucose tolerance remains unclear.

I agree that more studies are needed to assess the safety of Intermittent Fasting with women. I also think that this eating pattern is a good choice for anyone who wants to lose weight or control their diabetes.

The body speeds up its metabolism by a process called ketosis. Ketosis is an important part of the metabolic process that lets your body break down fat as fuel instead of breaking down muscle tissue, which could lead to obesity-related diseases like type 2 diabetes or heart diseases.

Normally, we eat food for energy that breaks down fats in our body that leads to fat burning and muscle growth. If your body doesn't get enough nutrients, it tends to use muscle tissue for breaking down fats. This leads to excessive loss of muscle mass that may lead to early aging.

Chapter 1. Why Intermittent Fasting for Women

Advantages and Benefits of Intermittent Fasting

Intermittent Fasting is a diet that involves fasting for limited periods. It means you also feast and eat a restricted number of times per day. In this section, we'll be discussing the advantages and benefits of Intermittent Fasting for women who are interested in living long, happy lives in one piece!

There are many reasons to consider Intermittent Fasting as an option to increase healthy longevity. The biggest reason is simply that it's not a new idea. Intermittent Fasting has been practiced for thousands of years by countries all over the world, and it just makes intuitive sense not to eat regularly. When we eat less frequently, we break down more slowly than when we're active in the day and rapidly digesting food at night.

Another benefit of Intermittent Fasting is weight loss. As we age, our metabolism slows down in certain areas, like the digestive tract. The body consumes energy more slowly when we're fasting, using it to digest food and keep us warm; so, for us to feel full, we have to eat less. If we take away the time needed to digest food, we can eat fewer calories and still feel full. The body also consumes energy more slowly when we eat every couple of hours. This extra energy is then used to repair our bodies rather than being stored as fat.

While I don't recommend aggressive dieting for you to lose pounds, Intermittent Fasting is a good way to turn down the volume on catabolic activity (breaking down body tissue) instead of increasing it.

There are many other benefits to Intermittent Fasting. Intermittent Fasting tends to improve your heart's health, as well as your brain. Your heart gets a break from working when you're not eating for 20+ hours each day, making it a better and healthier organ. The blood circulation in your brain is improved thanks to the effective movement of the muscles in your digestive tract, and this strengthens brain function! Having less work done on a day-to-day basis means better use of ATP (energy) and mitochondria (the energy powerhouses in cells).

Pay Attention to These Signs When Starting Intermittent Fasting (Potential Risk of Intermittent Fasting for Women)

1. Watch your caloric intake; if you are eating less than 1200 calories, you may not lose weight.
2. Include exercise in your days to help prevent muscle loss and the negative effects of aging on muscle tissue.
3. Have a plan for what type of Intermittent Fasting you will be doing (24-hour fasts, 18-hour fasts, etc.).
4. Regularly pay attention to how your body is feeling and adjust the schedule as needed for maximum results.
5. Talk to your doctor before beginning any new diet or exercise routine.

6. If you are interested in starting Intermittent Fasting to help with weight loss, heart health, or cognitive function, check out this part for help to get started (the benefits of Intermittent Fasting for Women).

7. If you are interested in trying a 24-hour fast, I suggest reading this first for tips. (Benefits of Intermittent Fasting for women).

8. Know that Intermittent Fasting is not just a tool to use with diet, but it can improve your life, prevent chronic diseases, and improve mental clarity (Intermittent Fasting Health Benefits for Women).

Chapter 2. Types of Intermittent Fasting

The 16:8 Method: Fast for 16 Hours Each Day

The 16:8 method is one of the most popular fasting diets out there. Simply put, it consists of fasting for 16 hours and eating during an 8-hour window. For instance, you fast from 1 pm until 9 pm, and then eat your next meal at 11 am the following day.

The 5:2 Diet: Fast for 2 Days per Week

This fasting diet limits you to a 500 calorie intake for 2 days each week. This will result in a significant weight loss, often 10 pounds or more.

Alternate-Day Fasting: Fast Every Other Day

Every other day, you eat nothing but non-caloric drinks, and on the days where you're eating, you're limited to 500 calories.

24-Hour Fast/One Meal a Day

Fasting for 24 hours, then eating one meal within a 12-hour window. Example: eating dinner at 6 pm and breakfast the next morning at 6 am.

Eat-Stop-Eat: Do a 24-Hour Fast, Once or Twice a Week

Many Intermittent Fasting programs suggest that you do a 24-hour fast once or twice a week. This approach is commonly called eat-stop-eat, and the idea is to retreat from eating food for 24 hours and then only take in water. Some of the benefits of this type of Intermittent Fasting are that it's easier on your digestive system as there are no solid foods for your body to break down, and it can jumpstart your weight loss. However, if you're doing this alone and not under the guidance of a certified professional, then we recommend you consult with them first before going through any fasting process alone. With this method, the healthiest and most ideal way to complete your fast would be during the night before you go to bed.

The Warrior Diet: Fast During the Day, Eat a Huge Meal at Night

This diet is best for people who can't imagine fasting for more than a couple of hours at a time. It's a simple idea: during the day, you eat nothing. No breakfast, no lunch, and no snacks. Just water (you can drink it anytime). Dinner is your one meal of the day—a big one.

Spontaneous Meal Skipping: Skip Meals When Convenient

The most common type of Intermittent Fasting is spontaneous meal skipping or 24-hour fast. Your goal on this program would be to not eat anything for a full 24 hours and then have a regular, healthy, nutritious meal when you're ready.

- **The Benefit:** this type of Fasting is that it gives your digestive system time off from working hard to break down food. It also stretches out the number of hours in which you could get your

16

required nutrients, which can be an issue with shorter types of Fasting because you might start starving before it's time for your next meal.

- **The Drawback:** the drawback to the spontaneous meal skipping type of Intermittent Fasting is that you will need to make sure you are getting enough calories to provide for your needs. This can be a challenge on a regular, healthy diet, but you can't let yourself get too hungry or risk overeating.

Choosing Your Intermittent Fasting Plan

Choosing your Intermittent Fasting plan should depend on your goals. If you want to lose weight, then it is best to stick with an Intermittent Fasting approach that involves fasts of 16 hours or more per day. On the other hand, if your goal is to improve cognitive function and cancer risk reduction, then you should choose an Intermittent Fasting plan that requires fasts of fewer than 16 hours per day.

Chapter 3. Mistakes to Avoid During Intermittent Fasting

Rushing into Intermittent Fasting

Rushing into Intermittent Fasting is a mistake many people make. It can be done, but there are some things to think about before jumping in head first. If your goal is weight loss, then Intermittent Fasting may not be the best course of action. Intermittent Fasting may not be for you if you have type 1 diabetes, type 2 diabetes, high blood pressure, or any other health condition where it's advised to eat regularly and monitor sugar levels throughout the day.

Choosing the Wrong Fasting Plan for Yourself

If you're an inexperienced intermittent faster, it's important to find a fasting plan that's suitable for your needs. If you're overweight or have a history of disordered eating, then try the 16:8 fasting plan, which entails limiting your daily intake to 12 hours from between dinner time until breakfast. If you're already healthy and only want to lose weight without too much effort, then choose the 24-hour fasting plan and eat all of your meals in an 8-hour window.

Not Drinking Enough and Drinking the Wrong Stuff

Not drinking enough and drinking the wrong stuff during the fasting period are two of the most common mistakes people make when doing intermittent Fasting. To avoid these mistakes, keep in mind these four important guidelines:

- Drink a full 8 ounces of water before you start fasting to help your body stay hydrated. Remember that coffee and tea count towards this 8-ounce amount, so if you want to drink them during your fast, then be sure to factor them into your total.
- Drink at least 8 ounces of water every hour during the fast.
- Drink at least 8 ounces of water immediately after you finish your extended fast.
- Resist the urge to drink other beverages during the fasting period. These include juice, tea, coffee, and alcohol.

People make the mistake of not drinking enough for several reasons: they forget to drink, they choose not to drink enough because it's inconvenient or uncomfortable, or they force themselves to stop drinking altogether because they think it will help them lose weight faster. It is true that you will lose weight faster if you have less fluid in your body, but only for two reasons: 1. if the extra fluid is fat, then it will be converted to ketones and excreted. 2. The body will draw upon stored liquids (i.e., your muscles) to maintain the appropriate volume of blood in your circulatory system. This is not unhealthy, but it is unnecessary weight loss (i.e., water loss).

Overeating When Fasting Ends

Overeating when fasting ends leads to weight gain, which defeats the whole purpose of fasting. We've compiled a list of mistakes you should avoid when Intermittent Fasting to keep your Fasting from undoing all your hard work.

- Start by eating a small meal before you begin your fast.
- Drink plenty of water and other fluids, like coffee or tea.
- Avoid high-fat foods that are slow to digest; eat lean protein instead.
- Don't go for an all-out binge when the fast is over; start with small snacks like salads and soups, then work up to larger meals as time goes on.
- Do not eat calorie-dense foods like meats, cheese, and butter.
- Do not gorge on food immediately after stopping fasting. It takes a while for your body to digest solid foods, so take your time.
- Avoid sugary foods that are packed with calories and fat since these slow down digestion.
- Fruits are high in sugar, but they're healthy. You can still eat these during a fast; just try to avoid the ones with added sugar or high fructose corn syrup. Stick to berries because they have less sugar than other fruits (and much more fiber).
- Limit the alcohol; alcohol adds empty calories and interferes with the fast.

- Caffeine is not a good idea because it can interfere with your body's ability to burn fat.

- Stay away from cheap chocolate bars that will spike your insulin levels and make you feel sick. Eat dark chocolate instead, or pick natural unsweetened cocoa as a healthy alternative if you like sweet treats.

- Avoid eating as many high fiber foods as possible, since they slow down your digestion and make you feel bloated. Try eating more whole grains, nuts, seeds, and vegetables during Intermittent Fasting.

Eating Too Much in the Fasting Window

This is a mistake because it will not only lead to caloric intake outside of the fasting window but also provide more nutrients to your cells so they can use them when you eat. This means your cells have to work harder than they would if you ate less and had the same number of calories in your fasting window.

Forcing It on Your Self

Just because you eat nothing for a certain period each day doesn't mean an eating disorder will just magically develop. If you're doing Intermittent Fasting correctly, your goal is not to starve yourself and deprive yourself of food; it's simply to eat less. Intermittent Fasting is designed to be a healthy weight-loss tool, so if you are also using it as a way to create anorexia or bulimia, that's not what this diet was designed for, and your results will be much worse than normal.

Not Paying Attention to the Nutrient Quality of the Foods

Not paying attention to the nutrient quality of the foods you eat, weight cycling, eating too big a breakfast, not drinking enough water. These are just some of the mistakes that can sabotage your efforts during Intermittent Fasting. Fortunately, we're here to give you some tried and tested pointers and show you exactly what you should do during Intermittent Fasting!

- Avoid snacks high in sugar or fat content (even if they're healthy). They will slow down any weight loss effort.
- Try and drink at least 2 liters of water per day. It will also hydrate your body and support a better metabolic rate for the time spent awake.
- Set aside one day each week where you break your fast with an "off" meal—often called a "cheat meal." It's hard to "cheat" on something you've never done before, but even if you're not fully committed to following the plan, some healthy grains or a small portion of lean meat would be a good blend of protein and fat for energy boost.

The most important way to lose weight is to burn more calories than you eat. To shed fat and prevent gaining back weight after your body has gotten back into "stubborn" mode, it's a good idea to consume 500-1,000 fewer calories per day than your normal intake. Your weight loss (or gain) will slow down as your metabolism settles into a new pace.

Restricting the Food Intake too Much

Restricting the food intake too much can be very harmful to your health. The length of the Intermittent Fasting is important to avoid these mistakes. When fasting for more than 18–22 hours can lead to ketosis, uncontrolled production of ketones in the body, which can lead to various health problems. However, when fasting for less than 18 hours, it won't lead to ketosis, and you can consume caffeine drinks when needed without worries.

Chapter 4. Food to Eat and Avoid in Intermittent Fasting

With all the health benefits of fasting on the rise, it is no surprise that a lot of people are looking for Intermittent Fasting. But what can you eat and what should be avoided? In this section, we will go through common questions for women in this age bracket.

We often think about exercise, sleep, and meditation as the easiest ways to lose weight. Intermittent Fasting offers an easy solution when it comes to weight loss, especially if you're struggling with things like obesity or diabetes risk factors. One thing, however, is not clear: what you should eat before you start intermittent fasting.

There has been a lot of advice on the internet about this topic. But surprisingly, there is very little science to back up any given diet. In fact, many different diets are advertised online as being perfect for women as they get older. But when we looked at those diets carefully, we discovered that they actually provide very little nutrition—all for little weight loss benefits. Which brings us to the real question: What should the women eat before intermittent fasting?

Intermittent Fasting for Women–What to Eat

The truth is that you don't have to do anything special to start an intermittent fast. The first step is simply to eat less and burn more calories than normal. This will force your body into a caloric deficit. With a caloric deficit, your body will be forced into fat storage mode, which is important because it is easier for it to burn fat than other sources of energy. This will help you lose weight faster.

Most women do not eat enough during the day. This can make it hard to start Intermittent Fasting because you will feel hungry all the time. It is important to keep this hunger in check so that you can continue with your fasts for a prolonged time. Here are some tips to help you get through your fasting period smoothly:

- **Keep a food journal!** This is especially important if you have never tried Intermittent Fasting before. By keeping track of what you were eating and drinking during your fasting periods, it will become easier for you to identify patterns that may not be working in your favor. These include foods that cause discomfort and those that help you get through a fasting period easier.

- **Increase your water intake!** This is one of the most important things you can do if you want to lose weight, but it is often ignored. Drinking water will help you lose a lot of water weight that might be difficult to shed when fasting. Water can also help your body digest food more effectively and make fat burning easier.

- **Eat more vegetables!** Vegetables are high in fiber, which helps the body burn fat and regulate hormones that can lead to weight loss. Also, many women do not eat enough vegetables, which leads to insufficient nutrition for their body–specifically for their metabolism. Eating more vegetables will ensure you get all the nutrients your body needs during a fasting period.

- **Eating the right food!** It can help you make the most out of Intermittent Fasting.

Intermittent Fasting for Women—What to Avoid

While eating or drinking certain foods can help you through your fast, some other foods and drinks will make things harder. Here are some suggestions of what you should avoid:

- **Caffeine:** It is a stimulant that makes it hard for your body to burn fat. Caffeine is found in tea, coffee, and energy drinks–most of which are consumed by women during the morning hours when they want to be productive. Caffeine is not good for your health and can make it difficult to complete a fast.

- **Alcohol:** Drinking alcohol reduces the effectiveness of Intermittent Fasting because alcohol causes an increase in insulin levels, which leads to increased fat storage. Alcohol also blocks nutrients from being absorbed by the body, meaning you may miss out on nutrients that can make it easier for you to lose weight. Too much caffeine or alcohol: both of these will inhibit fat burning during a fast.

- **Fries:** Most diets tell you to avoid fries if you want to lose weight, but that doesn't mean they should be completely avoided. However, when fasting, it is important to limit your intake of carbohydrates because they will prevent your body from burning fat and lead to increased hunger. Potatoes are high in carbohydrates (and therefore high in calories), so you must eat them with other vegetables and protein sources during a fast.

- If you suffer from celiac disease or gluten sensitivity, avoiding gluten can help you eliminate the symptoms of headaches, fatigue, and bad breath. It can also help you lose weight and boost your energy levels. You should get tested for celiac disease before going on a gluten-free diet; otherwise, you might experience weight gain rather than weight loss.

Also, if you are eating poorly, it might be hard to lose weight due to the extra pounds you are carrying around. If this is the case, consider making some lifestyle changes. This includes waking up earlier and going to bed later so that you can eat a healthy breakfast before starting your day and not binge during the evenings.

If you are following an Intermittent Fasting plan, it is best to consult with your doctor first before starting it so that he can give you a full assessment, including a blood test, hormone levels, and other health conditions. If you are experiencing some health symptoms while fasting, it is best to consult a doctor as soon as possible so that he can help you find the best treatment options for you.

Chapter 5. Intermittent Fasting Appetizers, Sides and Snacks Recipes

Starving in front of the fridge never felt so good! These appetizers, sides, and snacks are healthy and easy to make when you're on an Intermittent Fasting diet. In this section, we'll show you what kind of foods to eat before and after your fast so that you're satisfied without feeling deprived. With these recipes in hand, your only battle is with hunger. *Bon appétit!*

Cooking for an eating plan that involves fasting every day can be a challenge. Fasting can lead to weakness and headaches if not done correctly over time, but these recipes are designed specifically for those times when we have no food available to us because of our fasting schedule. The following recipes are designed to help you feel full and satisfied without feeling like you're on a diet. They're also designed for those with food allergies and those who need to be more conscious of their portion size.

1. Chicken Cordon Bleu

Preparation time: 5 minutes

Cooking time: 10 minutes

Servings: 4

The serving size is per tablespoon of chicken mixture only.

Ingredients:

- 1 pound skinless boneless chicken breast cut into bite-size pieces
- 1 stick string cheese (8 oz)
- 2 slices deli ham
- 1 egg

Directions:

1. Preheat oven to 350 degrees.
2. Line a baking sheet with parchment paper. Coat the chicken bites in egg and roll them in crushed pork rinds or bread crumbs to coat thoroughly. Place the chicken on the baking sheet and bake until cooked for about 10 minutes.
3. In a small bowl, melt the cheese in the microwave.
4. Spread half of it on a piece of ham. Cut off one corner of each piece of cheese to make "filling bags." Place one filled bag inside each chicken breast, then roll them up wraps and secure with a toothpick. Top with remaining cheese on top and roll back up.
   Note: To make an "all in one" low carb appetizer, prepare the chicken mixture as stated above, then top with sliced tomato and sliced avocado.

Nutrition:

- **Protein**: 71% 119
- **Fat**: 28% 49
- **Carbohydrates**: 1% 1

2. Cajun Chicken Fingers

Preparation time: 10 minutes

Cooking time: 8 minutes

Servings: 4

The serving size is per tablespoon of chicken mixture only.

Ingredients:

- 2 pounds skinless, boneless chicken breast cut into 1-inch pieces
- ¾ cup cheddar cheese, shredded
- ½ cup butter or bacon grease
- 1 tablespoon Cajun seasoning

Directions:

1. Preheat oven to 350 degrees. Melt butter in a large skillet over medium heat.
2. Add the chicken and cook until browned, about 5 minutes. Stir in Cajun seasoning and cook until well combined and slightly reduced, about 3 more minutes. Remove chicken from pan and set aside.
3. In the same pan over medium heat, add the cheese and stir until melted, about 3 more minutes.
4. Add the chicken back to the pan and mix well. Taste and add more seasoning if desired.

5. Microwave on 50% power for about 1 minute or until bubbly.

Note: To make an "all in one" low-carb appetizer, prepare the chicken mixture as stated above, then top with sliced tomato and sliced avocado.

Nutrition: (per ¼ cup)

- **Calories:** 6
- **Fat:** 0.5 g
- **Carbs:** 0 g
- **Protein:** 1 g

3. Pesto Stuffed Mushrooms

Preparation time: 5 minutes

Cooking time: 15 minutes

Servings: 4

The serving size is per tablespoon of chicken mixture only.

Ingredients:

- 1 pound mushrooms (any variety will do), stems trimmed
- 1 teaspoon cornstarch
- ½ teaspoon black pepper
- ¼ cup seasoned bread crumbs
- 3 tablespoons Parmesan or Parmigiano Reggiano cheese
- ½ cup chopped fresh basil
- ⅓ cup Italian pesto sauce

Directions:

1. Preheat oven to 350 degrees.
2. Line a baking sheet with foil. Place the mushrooms on the baking sheet and season with cornstarch and pepper. Top each mushroom half with the bread crumbs, cheese, and basil. Bake until tender, about 15 minutes.
3. In a small bowl, melt the cheese in the microwave. Spread half of it on a piece of basil, roll up wraps, and secure with a toothpick.

Top each half of the mushroom with the remaining cheese, then roll back up.

4. Serve hot.

Nutrition: (per ¼ cup)

- **Calories**: 6
- **Fat**: 0.2 g
- **Carbs**: 0.2 g
- **Protein**: 1 g

4. Kickin' Crab Cakes

Preparation time: 5 minutes

Cooking time: 15 minutes

Servings: 4

The serving size is per tablespoon of chicken mixture only.

Ingredients:

- 1 pound crabmeat (see notes), divided into two portions
- ½ cup mayonnaise
- 2 tablespoons Dijon mustard
- 1 tablespoon lemon juice
- 1 teaspoon seasoning salt (optional)
- 3 large celery stalks, thinly sliced ½ cup onion, minced
- 1 cup cooked green beans (about 1−1/2 cup)
- ⅓ cup chopped fresh parsley

Directions:

1. Preheat oven to 350 degrees.
2. In a medium-sized bowl, combine the crabmeat and half of the mayonnaise. Add the mustard and lemon juice. Combine well.
3. Line a baking sheet with foil. Place the remaining half of the mayonnaise in a small bowl, set it aside.

4. Bring the oven to 350 degrees.

5. In another medium bowl, combine salty with celery and onions. Toss to mix well. Dip your hands in water to prevent sticking and make 1" cakes of crab mixture. Place on baking sheet.

6. Bake for 10 minutes, then remove from oven and turn each crab cake over carefully using a spatula for non-stick surfaces or a metal spatula for stainless steel surfaces. Spread mayonnaise with green beans on one side of the crab cakes. Top with chopped parsley, bake an additional 5 minutes or until golden brown, or until heated through and crab is warmed all the way through. Serve with the extra green beans.

Nutrition:

- **Calories**: 58 calories
- **Total Fat**: 3.5 g (4% calories from fat)
- **Saturated Fat**: 12 g (55% calories from saturated fat)
- **Cholesterol**: 0.0 mgs (0% calories from fat)
- **Sodium**: 222.8 mgs (10% calories from sodium)
- **Carbohydrates**: 3 g (1% calories from carbs)
- **Fiber**: 0.5 g
- **Sugar**: 2 g
- **Protein**: 11.5 g

5. Quinoa Bowl

Preparation time: 10 minutes

Cooking time: 25 minutes

Servings: 2

Ingredients:

- 1 cup quinoa
- 1 banana
- 6 strawberries
- 2 cups water (coconut or regular)
- Cinnamon to taste (optional)
- Raspberries if desired (optional)
- Blueberries if desired (optional)

Directions:

1. Soak the quinoa overnight in the water and drain.
2. Add to a rice cooker with 2 cups of water and cook for 10 minutes.
3. Once cooked, add the strawberries, banana, cinnamon (optional), and raspberries/blueberries.
4. Continue adding water to the rice cooker as needed until ready to serve.
5. Stir and enjoy.

Nutrition:

- **Protein**: 15% 49 kcal
- **Fat**: 15% 47 kcal
- **Carbohydrates**: 70% 229 kcal

6. Spinach Salad with Muhammara

Preparation time: 10 minutes

Cooking time: 20 minutes

Servings: 4–6

Ingredients:

- 1 cup cooked quinoa
- ½ cup organic spinach, chopped
- 1 tablespoon extra virgin olive oil
- 3 to 4 tablespoons Muhammara
- 1 teaspoon balsamic vinegar or lemon juice Salt and pepper to taste

Directions:

1. Mix all ingredients until well combined.
2. Enjoy it with a mixture of whole foods from the produce section in your grocery store (avoid ingredients with high fructose corn syrup and sugar).

Nutrition:

- **Protein**: 13% 7 kcal
- **Fat**: 30% 15 kcal
- **Carbohydrates**: 57% 28 kcal

Chapter 6. Intermittent Fasting Poultry and Meat Recipes

7. Yogurt Chicken

Preparation time: 40 minutes

Cooking time: 15 minutes

Servings: 4

Ingredients:

- 1 pound chicken breast, boneless and skinless
- ½ cup plain Greek yogurt (non-fat)
- Juice from 1 lemon or lime
- 1 teaspoon dried oregano
- Salt and pepper to taste

Directions:

1. Cook chicken breasts in a skillet over medium heat with a little bit of olive oil for 2–3 minutes per side, or until chicken is cooked thoroughly and juices run clear. Remove from pan and let sit.
2. On the same pan, add in Greek yogurt, lemon or lime juice, oregano, and salt and pepper to taste. Mix well for about 10 minutes until the ½ cup of yogurt is melted, and the mixture is smooth.

3. Whisk back into the skillet as you return cooked chicken to the pan.

4. Cook for a couple more minutes until heated through.

5. Serve with rice or quinoa if desired.

Nutrition:

- **Calories:** 200
- **Protein**: 23.89 g
- **Fat**: 10.52 g
- **Carbohydrates**: 1.24 g

8. Blackened Tilapia with Mango Salsa

Preparation time: 30 minutes

Cooking time: 20 minutes

Servings: 4

Ingredients:

- 1 tilapia fillet (about 1/2 pound)
- 1/4 teaspoon paprika
- 1/4 teaspoon onion powder
- 1/4 teaspoon black pepper
- 1 mango, cubed (or more depending on size)
- Juice from 1 lime

Directions:

1. Preheat oven to 350 degrees.
2. Line a baking sheet with foil and place an oven-safe skillet or dish on top of the foil. Spray olive oil in the skillet and spread around evenly. Place tilapia on top of the skillet and sprinkle paprika, onion powder, and pepper over it.
3. Bake for 10–12 minutes, or until fish flakes easily with a fork.
4. Mix the cubed mango and lime juice in a bowl.

5. Once fish is removed from the oven, carefully remove the hot skillet/dish from underneath it. Top cooked fish with onions and mango salsa and serve with quinoa or rice if desired.

Nutrition:

- **Calories:** 32 kcal
- **Protein**: 5.92 g
- **Fat**: 0.53 g
- **Carbohydrates**: 1.24 g

9. Greek Chicken Salad

Preparation time: 25 minutes

Cooking time: 10 minutes

Servings: 4

Ingredients:

- 1 cup frozen or fresh spinach, chopped
- 2 cups cooked chicken chopped into small pieces (I like to use rotisserie chicken) 1/4 cup red onion, chopped
- 2 tomatoes
- diced 3 cucumbers
- diced 1 cup feta cheese
- 2 tbsp. lemon juice
- 3-4 tbsp. olive oil
- salt & pepper to taste
- 5 cups of your favorite salad greens

Directions:

1. Start by chopping your spinach, chicken, tomatoes, cucumbers and red onion.

2. Chop your cucumbers and tomatoes into small pieces.

3. Dice your red onion in small pieces, or chop it up very fine so no one will know there is a raw onion on their plate! You may want to use a vegetarian sour cream in place of the feta cheese for those vegetarians out there who do not eat meat or dairy products.

4. Chop your chicken into small pieces so that it is easier to eat with a fork and gets mixed up with the other ingredients in the salad easier!

.

5. Put spinach in processor to chop it up fine. Put spinach in small bowl and set aside.

6. Add your cucumbers, tomatoes, and red onion to the bowl to combine with the chicken, cheese, and dressing. This is your salad!

7. Top off your salad with the feta cheese and dressing of your choosing.

Nutrition:

- **Calories:** 21 kcal
- **Protein:** 2 g
- **Fat:** 0.33 g
- **Carbohydrates:** 3.17 g

10. Chicken Fajita Tacos with Avocado Sauce

Preparation time: 25 minutes (includes marinating time)

Cooking time: 20 minutes

Servings: 4

Ingredients:

- 2 whole-wheat tortillas
- 1 tablespoon olive oil
- 1/2 pound chicken breast, diced
- 1/2 yellow onion, chopped and sautéed in 1 tablespoon olive oil
- 1/4 cup low-fat sour cream
- 1 tablespoon chopped cilantro
- 2 tablespoons chopped scallions (white and green parts), also known as green onions
- 2 cups Spanish rice or 1/2 cup instant white rice
- 2 tablespoons sour cream
- 1 teaspoon chopped cilantro
- 3 tablespoons chopped scallions (white and green parts), also known as green onions
- 1 teaspoon garlic powder
- 1 orange

Directions:

1. First heat a skillet with 1 tablespoon of olive oil on medium-high heat. Add the diced chicken breast first, season lightly with salt, pepper, and garlic powder to taste. Cook until all sides are lightly browned. Then add 1/2 cup of chicken broth to deglaze (see notes). Cook for another 5 minutes or so; it will be slightly translucent but not fully cooked through yet. Remove the chicken from the pan and set it aside in a separate dish.

2. To the same pan, add another tablespoon of olive oil to the hot skillet. Add the onions, season with salt and pepper. Sautee until golden brown and remove from the pan. Remove all but 1 tablespoon of onion from the pan to use in the rice along with 1 cup of low sodium chicken broth.

3. In a medium saucepan, add 2 cups of water, 1 orange wedge (cut into quarters), and sliced grape tomatoes (set aside in a bowl). Bring water to a boil over high heat, once boiling lower heat, and simmer for 10 minutes or until tomatoes are softish but not fully cooked yet. Then pour onto rice mixture and mix.

4. Add 1/2 cup of cooked rice to the chicken mixture and mix thoroughly (see notes). Add salt and pepper to taste. Place fajita filling into warm tortillas. Top with sour cream, cilantro, scallions, avocado chunks, and thinly sliced grape tomatoes (see notes).

Notes: The garlic powder used is about 1 teaspoon. Rice has to cook for 20 minutes while covered with a lid at low heat. If you don't have an orange to use, as mentioned above, it will be ok to omit it or substitute orange juice or water instead of it, but the flavor won't be as prominent in the rice. Avocado has to be chopped into small chunks or slices to make them easier to mix. The scallion is about 1 tablespoon of chopped scallions. It is better if they are fresh but if you can't find them, just use 1 teaspoon of dried green onions instead.

In a separate bowl, add sour cream and cilantro and mix. Also, add the chopped green onions. The amount of chopped onion you use can be changed depending on your preference, but I would recommend about 1/4 cup or more for the rice, chicken filling, and sour cream mixture. The amount of sour cream you use can be changed depending on your preference.

Nutrition:

- **Calories:** 367
- **Protein**: 18.56 g
- **Fat**: 17.08 g
- **Carbohydrates**: 34.43 g

11. Chicken Breast with Black Bean Salsa

Preparation time: 10 minutes

Cooking time: 20 minutes (stovetop) or 6 minutes (Instant Pot)

Servings: 4-6 people depending on appetites and side dishes

Ingredients:

- 1 1/4 cups water or chicken stock (vegetable broth works great too!)
- 2 tablespoon olive oil, divided
- 1 cup onion, diced
- 1 medium jalapeno pepper (seeded and diced)
- 2 tablespoon garlic cloves, minced
- 1 can black beans, rinsed, and drained
- 2 chipotle peppers in adobo sauce, chopped
- 3 tablespoons fresh cilantro, chopped
- 2 Roma tomatoes, chopped
- 1/2 teaspoon salt
- 1 ½ pounds chicken breasts (boneless, skinless, and cut into 1–2 inch pieces)

Directions:

1. Place the black beans, chopped chipotle peppers, onion, cilantro, and garlic in a food processor or blender; pulse until smooth.

2. In your Instant Pot or on your stovetop: heat 1 tablespoon of olive oil over medium heat, then add the chicken in a single layer along with the salt and cook for about 4-6 minutes to brown all sides of the chicken. Remove cooked chicken to a separate plate and set aside; add remaining olive oil to the pot/skillet if needed and then add your onions and jalapeno pepper; cook for about 2 minutes until softened.

3. Stir in the salsa/sauce from the food processor or blender; cook for about 5 minutes until the sauce starts to thicken and coat the onions and pepper.

4. Add back in your chicken, tomatoes, and black beans; stir to combine all the ingredients.

5. Cover and set your Instant Pot on MANUAL (high pressure). Set the time to 6 minutes.

6. When your timer goes off, use the quick release method to release pressure. (You may have to do this in a few stages depending on your Instant Pot. If you are doing this on the stovetop, heat until boiling, then cover and reduce heat to low and simmer for about 15 minutes or until chicken is cooked through and tender.)

7. Remove the chicken to a serving bowl with some of the salsa/sauce; stir in cilantro just before serving. Serve with rice or tortillas, extra salsa/sauce, sour cream, and guacamole!

Nutrition:

- **Calories**: 203.9

- **Total Fat**: 6.3 g
- **Saturated Fat**: 1.2 g
- **Polyunsaturated Fat**: 1.5 g
- **Monounsaturated Fat**: 3.1 g
- **Cholesterol**: 69 mg
- Sodium: 697 mg
- **Potassium**: 438 mg
- **Carbohydrates**: 10.2 g
- **Fiber**: 2.7 g
- **Sugar**: 3.2 g
- **Protein**: 28.6 g

12. Buffalo Chicken and Blue Cheese Stuffed Poblano Peppers

Preparation time: 15 minutes (includes marinating time)

Cooking time: 25 minutes

Servings: 4

Ingredients:

- 2 poblano peppers, halved and deseeded
- 1 cup cooked chicken, cut into 1" pieces
- 2 tablespoons hot sauce
- 4 ounces cream cheese
- 1/2 cup buffalo sauce
- 4 ounces blue cheese crumbles
- 3/4 cup blue cheese dressing
- Salt and pepper to taste

Directions:

1. Place the poblano peppers on a baking sheet. Broil on high for 8–10 minutes or until skin is charred.
2. Remove from the oven and place in a bag. Let them steam for 5 minutes, and then peel off the skin.
3. In a medium mixing bowl, combine the chicken with hot sauce and cream cheese. Stir to combine.

4. Add in buffalo sauce and mix well. Spread the mixture evenly on the inside of the peppers, making sure to not overfill. Sprinkle with blue cheese crumbles, then drizzle with blue cheese dressing. Season with salt and pepper to taste.

5. Serve immediately or refrigerate until ready to eat!

Nutrition:

- **Calories:** 396
- **Protein:** 9.65 g
- **Fat:** 33.37 g
- **Carbohydrates:** 14.62 g

Chapter 7. Intermittent Fasting Salad and Soups Recipe

13. Warm Salmon and Asparagus Salad

Servings: 4

Preparation time: 10 minutes

Cooking time: 8 minutes

Make this warm salmon and asparagus salad on a cool summer night. It is full of clean flavors, bright colors, and tons of crunchy texture. This is the epitome of clean eating. The honey Greek yogurt dressing perfectly coats the salmon. That, combined with the crunchy asparagus and sweet red onion, makes this salad an explosion of deliciousness in your mouth. The vinaigrette is easy to make, and the rest of the salad comes together in no time.

Ingredients:

- 1/2 pound salmon
- 1 tablespoon olive oil, divided use
- 1 teaspoon dried basil leaves, divided use
- 6 spears asparagus (about 1 cup) cut into 2-inch pieces—remove any tough ends or woody part of the stalk

- Salt to taste (optional)—you may not need any depending on how salty your dressing is
- 1/3 cup honey flavored Greek yogurt
- 1 teaspoon lemon juice (about 1 tablespoon lemon juice)—if you don't have the juice, add a little olive oil to get it the right consistency

For the Vinaigrette:

- 2 tablespoons olive oil (or canola, or vegetable oil)
- 2 teaspoons white vinegar (or unseasoned rice vinegar) or apple cider vinegar—use your favorite! You can replace this with a splash of water as well. It's also good without! You can see which one I prefer in this article. Start reading at the first paragraph! This is where I recommend using water and not vinegar.
- 1 tablespoon honey (or simple syrup or brown sugar)
- ½ teaspoon dried basil leaves (optional)

Directions:

1. In a small bowl, mix the honey, olive oil, vinegar or water, and basil leaves. If you are using water instead of vinegar, add about ½ teaspoon of olive oil at this time. The mixture should be a little runny but not too thin like water. This dressing will coat the asparagus nicely. Whisk it until well combined. Set aside for later use while cooking salmon and asparagus.

2. Place the salmon in a large bowl and drizzle with 1 teaspoon of olive oil. Season with salt and pepper to taste. Add the red onion slices on top of the salmon.

3. Use a bamboo or metal skewer to poke holes in the salmon throughout its body, being careful not to pierce too deep into the meat itself so that they don't increase in size or fall apart while cooking.

4. Preheat the oven to 400°F, and place a rack in the upper-middle section of the oven. Place a medium-sized skillet on the stove on high heat and allow it to get hot enough for you to feel some heat off the pan when you hold your hand an inch or so away from it. Place salmon skin-side down in the skillet, placing asparagus around salmon pieces. Add 1/2 tablespoon of oil on top of the salmon (you can use any type of oil) and sear each piece for approximately 2−3 minutes per side. Place skillet with asparagus and salmon into the oven for 4−5 minutes until fish has reached the desired doneness by using a kitchen thermometer.

5. Remove skillet from oven and allow to cool for 4−5 minutes. Then, use a butter knife or spatula to remove the salmon and asparagus onto a large plate (be careful because it will be hot!). Serve with honey Greek yogurt sauce over the top of each piece of salmon. Drizzle sauce evenly all over salmon. Don't be shy about it! You can also add some asparagus on the side for added crunch and texture.

Nutrition:

- **Calories:** 135
- **Protein**: 12.56 g
- **Fat**: 8.59 g
- **Carbohydrates**: 1.23 g

14. Honey Garlic Shrimp Salad

Servings: 4

Preparation time: 5 minutes

Cooking time: 15 minutes

This recipe is so easy to make and tastes delicious. You can use fresh shrimp or cooked shrimp as well. What's nice is that it's also a great way to get kids involved with the cooking process. Instead of buying pre-cooked shrimp, you can prepare this dish using your hand-picked fresh ones from your local farmer's market. This salad is crunchy, sweet, and refreshingly tasty.

Ingredients:

- 2 tablespoons oil (your choice)
- 1 pound shrimp, peeled and deveined
- 1 teaspoon salt or more per taste
- ½ teaspoon ground black pepper per taste. You can use white pepper if you like. It has a nice spicy kick to it! This recipe works well with either one. (I prefer white pepper)–be careful though, it can easily overpower the salad and leave your mouth on fire! So, start with small amounts! You can always add more later if you wish. (But 1/2 teaspoon should be good for most people)
- 1/2 cup honey
- 2 tablespoons soy sauce

- 1 tablespoon garlic oil or minced garlic (I prefer minced garlic)
- 4 cups lettuce, chopped (iceberg lettuce is a great one to use for this recipe) or Romaine lettuce, chopped. You can use any type of lettuce that you like, but iceberg tastes the best for me in this recipe. It's also hard to overcook. Other types of lettuce are more delicate and can easily get soggy if they are heated too long in the microwave. This is why I usually opt for using iceberg instead.
- ½ green or red bell pepper, chopped finely
- 1/4 cups cilantro, chopped finely
- 1/4 cup scallions, chopped finely
- 1 large carrot, shredded (or more if you like)

Directions:

1. Heat oil in a large pan on medium/high heat. Once it is hot and sizzling—toss in shrimp.
2. Sprinkle with salt and pepper and turn the shrimp over after approximately 30 seconds to a minute to have both sides of the shrimp become seared nicely.
3. Toss in the honey and soy sauce into the pan with the shrimp when it turns a caramel color—about 2 minutes total cooking time per side.
4. When either the soy sauce or honey starts to thicken, use a spatula to flip the shrimp and make sure not to burn it by turning it quickly.

5. Turn off the heat and add the garlic oil or minced garlic in. Toss again for 2−3 seconds.

6. Serve immediately in a salad bowl topped with your favorite types of lettuce (lettuce will be hard to eat if you overcook it) and garnished with cilantro and scallions.

This recipe made 6 large salads that all yield about 4 cups of each— perfect for lunch or dinner for one person! But you can easily double or even triple the recipe if you are feeding more than one person. This is an incredibly simple meal that will not disappoint. As mentioned, this recipe could also easily be doubled for extra servings or tripled if you need to feed a larger group.

Nutrition:

- **Calories:** 377
- **Protein**: 25.12 g
- **Fat**: 13.39 g
- **Carbohydrates**: 41.41 g

15. Honey Garlic Shrimp in Lettuce Bowls

Servings: 3

Preparation time: 5 mins

Cooking time: 10 mins

Total time: 15 mins

This Honey Garlic Shrimp in Lettuce Bowls is an incredibly low-carb meal that is perfect for lunch and dinner! Gluten-free, vegan, and paleo-friendly.

Ingredients:

- 3 cups shredded lettuce
- 1 tablespoon sesame oil
- 1 teaspoon fresh ginger, grated (or minced)
- 1 tablespoon garlic, minced
- 3 cups broccoli florets, chopped into bite-sized pieces
- 12 ounces raw shrimp (tails removed), cut into small chunks (about 1 inch long)

For the sauce:

- ½ cup light soy sauce or tamari (gluten-free)
- ¼ cup honey
- 2 tablespoons fresh orange juice

- 1 teaspoon sriracha sauce

Directions:

1. Thaw and chop the shrimp into small chunks and set aside.
2. Heat the sesame oil over medium-high heat in a nonstick pan. Stir fry the broccoli florets for 2 minutes and add the shrimp at the last minute, until cooked (about 1−2 minutes).
3. Combine all sauce ingredients in a small bowl and set aside.
4. Place about 3 cups of shredded lettuce into 3 bowls.
5. Add the stir-fried shrimp and veggies into the lettuce bowls and top with garlic sauce before serving.

Nutrition:

- **Calories**: 339 kcal
- **Fat**: 9 g
- **Carbohydrates**: 45 g
- **Sugar**: 24 g
- **Sodium**: 1646 mg
- **Fiber**: 2 g
- **Protein**: 31 g
- **Cholesterol**: 164 mg

16. Chicken Potato Carrot Soup

Servings: 3

Preparation time: 15 minutes

Cooking time: 30 minutes

Ingredients:

- 1 teaspoon olive oil
- 6 cups chicken broth
- 2 cups chicken breast, cooked and shredded
- 2 russet potatoes, peeled and diced
- 6 carrots, peeled and chopped
- ¼ cup diced celery
- 1/3 cup onion, chopped
- 1 cup water
- ½ teaspoon salt
- ¼ teaspoon freshly ground pepper
- Croutons for topping (optional)

Directions:

1. Heat the oil in a large saucepan over medium-high heat. Cook the onion and celery until the onions are translucent.
2. Add the broth and potatoes to the pan.

3. Add in the chicken breast, carrots, salt, and pepper. Bring to a boil.
4. Reduce heat and simmer, covered for 20–30 minutes or until the potatoes are tender.
5. Blend in the soup-blender (or food processor) until smooth.
6. Add more broth if you'd like a super creamy soup. Serve with croutons and enjoy!

Nutrition:

- **Calories:** 1177
- **Protein**: 139.28 g
- **Fat**: 38.56 g
- **Carbohydrates**: 61.26 g

17. Chilled Avocado Soup Recipe

Preparation time: 5 minutes

Cooking time: 10 minutes

Servings: 2

Ingredients:

- 3 ripe avocados
- 1 can full-fat organic coconut milk
- 1 small onion, chopped (optional)
- ½ cup fresh basil or basil pesto
- ¼ cup olive oil
- ¼ teaspoon sea salt and pepper to taste

Directions:

1. In your blender or food processor, add your avocado, olive oil, basil, salt, and pepper until you achieve a puree. This will require some blending or pulsing if using a blender.
2. In a bowl, add your puree to the rest of the ingredients listed and stir well. Cover with lid and place in the fridge for at least 8 hours (overnight is best).
3. Top with fresh basil and cracked pepper, then dig in! This soup is much like a chicken noodle, but it has fewer noodles and more

vegetables. It makes a great lunch and takes less than half an hour to make.

Nutrition:

- **Calories:** 739 kcal
- **Protein**: 6.72 g
- **Fat**: 71.28 g
- **Carbohydrates**: 29.68 g

18. Vegetable Soup

Preparation time: 15 minutes

Cooking time: 30 minutes

Servings: 6−8

Ingredients:

- 1 tablespoon olive oil, plus more for drizzling
- 2 minced garlic cloves
- 1 large onion diced
- 2 celery stalks chopped
- 3 carrots chopped into rounds or chunks
- 1 can crushed tomatoes (28 ounces) (1 pound 10 ounces) or 5 cups peeled and chopped fresh tomatoes. It can also be made with 8 cups of mashed cooked potato or pumpkin with juice added
- 8 cups spinach or kale
- 1 package sliced mushrooms (8 ounces). It can also be replaced with fresh mushrooms
- 1 package frozen lima beans (8 ounces) or 1 can drain and rinse
- 1 package fresh green peas (8 ounces). It can also be frozen and thawed for a few minutes to let them heat up

NOTE: Other vegetables may be used according to your taste.

Directions:

1. Boil a large pot of water (6–8 quarts); place spinach or kale into boiling water until wilted; drain in a colander.
2. Heat oil in a large pot, add onions, garlic, and sauté for about 10 minutes until it turns brown.
3. Add carrots, celery and continue cooking for another 10 minutes until carrots are slightly softened. Add canned crushed tomatoes or fresh tomatoes and mix well.
4. Add the spinach (avoid stems if possible) and the mushrooms.

Note: It can be replaced by fresh mushrooms and frozen lima beans.

5. Cover and cook on medium-low heat for about 30 to 40 minutes until potatoes are cooked through or the pasta is done, which takes the same amount of time depending on the type of pasta used.
6. Add salt and pepper to taste.

Nutrition:

- **Calories:** 117 kcal
- **Protein**: 5.76 g
- **Fat**: 2.36 g
- **Carbohydrates**: 20.21 g

Chapter 8. Intermittent Fasting Fish and Seafood Recipes

19. Grilled Tuna with Avocado

Preparation time: 15 minutes

Cooking time: 15 minutes

Servings: 4

Ingredients:

- 4 6-ounce ahi tuna fillets
- Extra virgin olive oil for brushing on the grill
- Sea salt flakes or coarse sea salt, to taste
- Black pepper, freshly ground, to taste
- 1 large ripe avocado
- Salt and pepper drizzle over the top before serving (optional)
- Foil-wrapped grill packet with vegetables (optional)

Directions:

1. Grill each side until browned but still soft in the center. Grilling fillets on the bone is the best way to maintain a tender texture. The skin tends to be dry, so removing it before grilling is not a

necessity. If you are using an outdoor grill, remove skin and cut fillets into steaks.

2. Preheat grill on high heat for 10 minutes or until it is hot enough to leave your hand over it for 3−4 seconds.

3. Brush each side of the tuna with olive oil and sprinkle with sea salt flakes or coarse salt and freshly ground pepper to taste.

4. Place foil-wrapped vegetables and/or fish packet on the grill. Grill each side for 5−8 minutes until browned but still soft in the center of ahi tuna steaks. (Cooking time depends on your grill.)

5. Move your hand over the grill about 3−4 inches above the surface and check for doneness.

6. When done, remove from heat and serve tuna as-is or with desired toppings.

7. To cut tuna steaks, hold with tongs and run a knife down the center until cooked through.

8. Serve alongside avocado slices or sprinkle sea salt flakes on top before serving simply for additional flavor. Top with a little black pepper just before serving for an added kick.

To enjoy grilled tuna, you can also serve it over a bed of lettuce with a bit of mayo dressing. Our favorite dressing is to blend one avocado with a dash of sea salt, black pepper, and lime juice.

Nutrition:

- **Calories:** 133 kcal
- **Protein**: 11.67 g

- **Fat**: 7.62 g
- **Carbohydrates**: 5.72 g

20. Smoked Fish Dip

Inspired by the idea of smoked salmon dip, this recipe utilizes the smoky flavor of trout or salmon in a white cheese dip. Use sour cream and cream cheese as your base for this homemade smoked fish dip. It may be used as an appetizer for crackers or raw vegetables or served with crackers and chips alongside burgers or sandwiches.

Preparation time: 20 minutes

Cooking time: 10 minutes

Servings: 2

Ingredients:

- 1/2 cup light cream cheese, softened
- 1/4 cup sour cream, or plain yogurt (may substitute mayonnaise)
- 5 ounces smoked trout or salmon, finely chopped
- 3 tablespoons finely chopped green onion (white and green parts)
- 1 tablespoon lemon juice from ¼-inch thick lemon peel; to taste. A pinch of sugar is good too. Salt and pepper to taste.
- 4 hard boiled eggs, peeled and sliced thin for garnish (may use 1-2 small jarred pickles instead). Minced chives for garnish.

Directions:

1. Place smoked trout and cream cheese into food processor or a blender. Pulse until well blended (do not over-mix).
2. Add the chopped egg whites, yogurt/mayonnaise, salt, pepper and lemon juice to taste.

3. Refrigerate if not serving immediately. If freezing, do so in freezer-safe containers.

Good with whole grain crackers and other appetizers/snacks.

Nutrition:

- **Calories:** 124 kcal
- **Protein**: 3.18 g
- **Fat**: 11.64 g
- **Carbohydrates**: 2.02 g

21. Smoked Salmon Sandwiches

Bring out the sophistication of smoked salmon by serving on an open-faced bagel sandwich. The cream cheese and chives add color to the overall presentation while enhancing the flavor of this delicious meal. Serve and garnish with tomato slices and fresh cucumber slices for added flair and flavor.

Preparation time: 20 minutes

Cooking time: 10 minutes

Servings: 2

Ingredients:

- Two 8-ounce packages (total) smoked salmon, cut into 12 slices
- 1 bottle Zesty Italian dressing (16 oz.)
- Four slices whole-wheat bread, lightly toasted with crusts removed and cut in half like a hamburger bun, about 1/2 inch thick. Or you can use two 7-ounce loaves of freshly baked homemade bread.
- Optional ingredients for sandwiches: Two tablespoons cream cheese spread. Two teaspoons lemon juice. One medium red onion, thinly sliced into rounds. Six caper berries, drained and rinsed. One teaspoon dried dill weed or one tablespoon chopped fresh dill weed.

Directions:

1. Arrange the salmon slices on four pieces of bread.

2. Spoon a heaping tablespoon of dressing on top of each piece of bread and spread it evenly to cover the salmon. Top the sandwich with optional ingredients, if you like. Try to avoid making a mess with the lemon juice and cream cheese or else it will make it difficult to eat the sandwich. If you're spreading lemon juice and/or cream cheese on your sandwich, be sure to use a knife rather than your hands. You wouldn't want your salmon-eating gloves to lose their scent!

3. Serve immediately while fresh ingredients are still moist and delicious.

Nutrition:

- **Calories:** 124 kcal
- **Protein**: 5.08 g
- **Fat**: 0.77 g
- **Carbohydrates**: 24.32 g

22. Butternut Squash Soup with Cinnamon Croutons

Preparation time: 20 minutes

Cooking time: 40 minutes

Servings: 2

Ingredients:

- 1 butternut squash, peeled and diced
- 1/2 onion, finely chopped
- 3 cloves garlic, minced
- 2 qts vegetable broth or water
- 4 tsp salt or to taste
- pepper to taste (optional)
- vegetable oil for frying croutons (optional)
- Chopped parsley for garnish (optional)

Directions:

1. Heat a large pot of salted water over high heat until boiling. Add the squash and onion, stirring occasionally with a wooden spoon until tender - about 10 minutes. Drain and set aside. Return the pot to high heat with some vegetable oil. Add the vegetables and fry until golden-brown, stirring frequently. Add the garlic and vegetable broth. Season with salt and pepper as desired.

2. Combine the ingredients in a blender (or use an immersion blender). Puree until very smooth, then pour back into the pot (over low heat), stir and heat through. Ladle into soup bowls and garnish with fresh parsley sprigs if desired. Serve with cinnamon croutons on top or on the side.

Nutrition:

- **Calories:** 44 kcal
- **Protein:** 1.25 g
- **Fat:** 0.14 g
- **Carbohydrates:** 10.62 g

23. Mediterranean Chickpea Soup with Red Bell Pepper and Basil

Preparation time: 20 minutes

Cooking time: 40 minutes

Servings: 4

Ingredients:

- 1 tbsp. extra virgin olive oil (EVOO)
- 1/2 tsp. dried red pepper flakes, plus more for garnish (optional)
- 4 cups chicken or vegetable broth, divided
- 2 cans (14 1/2 oz.) diced tomatoes with juice *see note below the recipe box for other suggestions on what to add here if you don't have tomato cans on hand.
- 5 cups cooked chickpeas (about 2 cans)
- 1 large shallot, chopped
- 3 cloves garlic, finely chopped
- 1/4 cup fresh basil, finely chopped (about 1 tbsp.)
- 8 oz. Greek yogurt (your choice of flavor or a combination...we like plain and flavored at the same time!)
- 1/4 tsp. sea salt ½ tsp. black pepper 1 tbsp. extra virgin olive oil

Directions:

1. In a medium pot over medium heat, add EVOO and red pepper flakes. Saute until the pepper is fragrant and the EVOO glistens. Next add the broth, tomatoes (if you choose not to use tomato cans...see notes below the recipe box), chickpeas, shallot, garlic and basil. Stir and bring to a boil. Reduce heat and simmer until shallots are translucent - about 15 minutes.

2. Using an immersion blender, blend the soup in the pot or transfer to a traditional blender in small batches. Blend until you reach your desired consistency.*

3. Taste and season with salt/pepper if needed, garnish with more red pepper flakes, if desired and serve with a dollop of yogurt to garnish.

*When blending, use caution because you don't want to push the soup too much and make it too smooth. You want to have a little texture so that it can stand up in the bowls and look like a hearty bowl of soup!

Other suggestions: Add celery, carrots, different pasta or rice noodles instead of chickpeas

*** We prefer canned tomatoes but if you don't feel like using cans right now or if you're out of these options...enjoy this soup with your favorite tomatoes (canned packed in water) and minced fresh garlic.

If not using tomato cans...place chicken broth in sauce pan over medium heat. Add onion and chopped garlic and saute until tender. Add canned tomatoes and cook for a few minutes. Add chickpeas, basil, tomatoes with juice, salt and pepper to taste.

Notes: This recipe is gluten-free and vegetarian. If you'd like to make it vegan, simply use vegetable broth and olive oil instead of chicken broth/meat.

Nutrition:

- **Calories:** 107
- **Protein**: 5.19 g
- **Fat**: 1.69 g
- **Carbohydrates**: 19.29 g

24. Creamy Cauliflower Soup with Crispy Fried Shallots

Preparation time: 15 minutes

Cooking time: 30 minutes

Servings: 4

Ingredients:

- 1 head cauliflower
- 2 cups vegetable broth
- 1 can coconut milk
- 1 shallot
- olive oil for frying

Directions:

1. Trim the greens off the cauliflower and chop it into chunks. Fill a pot with water and bring to boil over high heat. When boiling, add the cauliflower chunks and simmer for about 10-12 minutes until soft enough to pass through a sieve or food mill. Drain the cauliflower, reserving 1 cup of the cooking liquid, then transfer to a blender or food processor. Process until smooth. Set aside.

2. In a large saucepan over medium heat, pour in the vegetable stock and coconut milk. Heat until just simmering, then remove from heat and set aside.

3. Slice the shallot down to 1/3 its diameter then finely mince it. Pour about 1 inch of oil into a sauté pan over medium-high heat (the shallots will splatter if you use too little oil). When hot, carefully add the sliced shallots and fry them for 2 minutes until they turn light golden brown. Remove with a slotted spoon and drain on paper towels. Pour out the oil, then return the pan to medium-high heat. When hot, add about 1 tablespoon of olive oil, then add the minced shallot. Saute for another 2 minutes until the shallot turns golden brown. Drain on paper towels, then set aside.

4. To serve, pour the soup into 4 bowls over a few pieces of fried shallots.

Nutrition:

- **Calories:** 1
- **Protein**: 0.05 g
- **Fat**: 0 g
- **Carbohydrates**: 0.25 g

Chapter 9. Eating and Training: The Best Exercise Routine for Longevity

While exercise is an important aspect of maintaining your health, it can be difficult to know which exercises are best for you. Workout routines vary depending on your goals and fitness level. This will give a general idea of what might be the best workout routine for you.

If we are to achieve the goal of lifelong health, we must properly maintain our bodies by being physically active. Moreover, as we age, our bodies grow weaker and less resilient, so it's necessary to introduce physical activity into our lifestyle from a young age—otherwise, this process will become that much harder later in life when muscle tissue is broken down with age instead of built up from vigorous activity during youth.

To start, the most important thing to remember is that exercise should not be only about working out. It's about more than just moving around but also eating well and maintaining a healthy lifestyle. You should start by including these three pillars into your daily routine: eating well, getting regular exercise, and maintaining a healthy diet.

Eating well is essential for you to maintain a healthy body, as it is the main source of energy for you. If you are not eating enough calories or your diet lacks nutrients and vitamins, your body will not be able to perform the tasks it needs to do for you. You should eat seven small meals throughout the day instead of 3 large ones (this means 7 times smaller portions per meal). For example, let's say you need around 2,000 calories per day (how many calories you need depends on your gender, age, and weight). Eating seven meals a day will give you around 350 calories per meal. That means that 7 x 350 = 2,100 calories for the whole day.

Your diet should consist mainly of fresh food from your local supermarket or farmer's market. Processed foods are usually high in salt, sugar, and fat, so it's best to avoid them in favor of fresh, healthy food instead. Besides that, you should also make sure that the meat and fish you are eating are fresh and not frozen, as this can deplete your body of vitamins over time due to freezing processes. Here are five simple tips to help you eat well:

- **Eat a variety of fruits and vegetables!** Try and eat a minimum of 5 portions of fruit (this is equivalent to 1 piece at least) and 3 portions of vegetables. This will give you a balance between nutrients and vitamins so your body can stay healthy all the time. Experts say that monounsaturated fats from avocados, nuts, olive oil, or fish will help you lower your risks for diseases such as cancer, heart disease ordiabetes.

- **Drink a lot of water!** If you aren't drinking enough water, then it can cause dehydration, which can be dangerous for your health. Water helps your body cleanse itself from harmful toxins and makes you feel full, so it should be your number one food group.

85

- **Eat lean meats and fish (avoid fatty meat)!** Lean meats and fish are a great source of protein, iron, zinc, and omega 3. These nutrients are essential to help support the biological functions of the human body and will help in preventing diseases. A study published in the American Journal of Clinical Nutrition found that men that eat fish at least 2 times a week have a 25% lower risk of heart disease than those that don't eat any fish at all.

- **Drink herbal tea (avoid caffeine)!** Caffeine can be addictive and can cause your body to lose sleep. Many herbal teas are available at your local supermarket or online. For example, chamomile tea is good for calming down and helping you relax. Water helps your body get rid of harmful toxins more effectively while enjoying the great taste of your favorite teas.

- **Exercise!** This is not a tip but rather a necessity if you want to stay healthy. It's important to exercise regularly as it will help you stay mentally and physically healthy throughout your life and improve the quality of your life as well. Doctors recommend at least 150 minutes per week of moderate-intensity exercise or 75 minutes per week of vigorous-intensity exercise. To help you achieve this, you can do a combination of aerobic exercises such as jogging, swimming, or cycling and weight training exercises such as lifting weights or doing the bench press.

- **Supplementation!** It is also important to keep your body healthy and fight disease. Supplements allow you to get the nutrients and vitamins that you would not get from solely consuming food, which in turn helps your body function better. For example, fish oil is known to help prevent heart disease, and vitamin C helps the body resist colds and infections. There are also plenty of other supplements that you can purchase, for example, creatine or amino acids.

For a healthy and pleasurable life, it is essential to make exercise a part of your routine, as it will help you manage your daily stress and anxiety, which in turn will help you live a better life. Being active is more than just working out; it's about eating well, drinking water, and getting enough sleep to support your body. Thanks to the new research, we now know that there are many ways to incorporate physical activity into our lifestyle, however seeing as exercise is not on everyone's list of priorities, here are five easy exercises you can do anywhere anytime to stay fit:

- **Exercise while you watch TV!** Instead of just sitting on the couch or chair, try doing sets of squats while you watch your favorite TV show. This will tone your legs and increase your leg power which will help you when walking upstairs.

- **Exercise while you walk!** Instead of just walking from place to place, try to walk faster and do a quick exercise such as waving your arms around (make sure others can't see that!) or putting one foot behind the other and swinging it towards the front without touching the ground. It should not take long before you start sweating, and once again, it's a great way to tone up those legs!

- **Exercise while you wait!** Instead of just standing in the queue, do some sets of squats or push-ups while waiting for your turn.

- **Exercise on the toilet!** When you feel like doing a little dance to pass the time, try to do squats instead of just rocking your hips. To make it more challenging, try to hold a small weight up or even roll a dice at the same time! It's a great way to tone up those abs as well as raising your heart rate and blood pressure.

- **Exercise while you wait for the bus!** Instead of just standing in the queue, walk on to the bus. By doing so, you will be burning some calories, and with a little bit of luck, you might meet someone close by who is also taking up the challenge!

The idea of sitting down at a computer to watch your favorite TV shows or films is not ideal when it comes to your health. Working out while watching TV can help you achieve better results because it will keep your heart rate up and will help burn more calories than just sitting on your couch. Adding one or two super easy exercises to your daily routine can drastically improve your look and overall health. So go ahead and put your headphones on and get ready to exercise!

If you're looking for a more advanced workout, check out the Sadie Fikri Extreme Abs Workout! Use this to tone up your body and see results even faster. The Sadie Fikri Extreme Abs Workout is one of the best ways to get fit at home. Watch her videos and try it out yourself! She will show you how it's done.

How to Lose Fat without Exercising?

The secret to losing those stubborn pounds and losing that extra fat off your body is to eat a proper diet. In other words, if you want to lose weight, then you need to stop eating junk foods and start eating healthy foods. However, this will be very difficult for most people, as most of us are used to eating what we want all the time. But there's an easy trick that will help you lose weight, "Cut out the soda."

Cut out all the sodas like cola, lemonade, and other soft drinks. If you want to lose weight without exercising, then you'll have to give up all the soft drinks. This is because these soft drinks contain a lot of sugar, and the main source of sugar in our diet comes from soda. So, cutting out soda will not only help you lose weight but will also help you live a healthier life!

In this book you find recipes and tips that will provide you with high-impact nutrition that makes it easier for your body to break down and burn fat. I know that's a bit confusing, so let's clear it up a bit more! To "Break Down Fat" is to make it easier for your body to burn fat. You must create diet plans and foods that will help your body reach this goal of burning fat. To "Burn Fat" is to boost your metabolism so that your body can lose weight. So, you must create diet plans and foods that will help your body reach this goal.

Chapter 10. How to Overcome Down Moments in Intermittent Fasting

Start the Fast After Dinner

- Start the fast after dinner and break the fast in the morning.
- Stay away from drinks like caffeinated tea, coffee, and black tea or green tea.
- Do not drink alcohol during this time of day.
- Avoid foods with a lot of sugars like candy or desserts as well as refined grains like white bread, rice, pasta, and many bowls of cereal.
- Eat healthy fats such as avocados, olive oil, and nuts to help with satiety (feeling full) during the fasting period.
- Eat a huge bowl of fruit or vegetable salad after breaking the fast.
- Do not eat large meals during the fast. Stay away from salty and processed foods like chips, pretzels, crackers, crisps, bagels, and cookies.
- Make sure to drink at least 8 glasses of water per day since dehydration can impair fasting results.
- The fasting process should start around noon so you can take advantage of the night hours for sleep to replenish your tissues, whereas you will be more active during the daytime.

- Avoid fried foods and replace them with healthier options like grilled foods, baked foods, poached or roasted meats, and fish.

- Do not drink beverages containing calcium, as it will interfere with the fasting process. You can have tea, but no milk, since it contains sugars and stimulants that are counter-productive to fasting.

- Eat raw vegetables instead of cooked vegetables during the fast.

- Try to combine fasting with exercise or a brisk walk for long periods (30 to 60 minutes).

- Avoid taking naps and gradually increase your sleeping time if interrupted between days.

- The fasting process may take as much as 12 hours from midnight until noon the following day.

- If you feel like you want to eat, you may do so but stop eating as soon as you feel full and drink at least 16 fluid ounces of water at that time (Your water intake should not exceed 64 ounces per day since it might interfere with the results).

Eat More Satisfying Meals

Eat more satisfying meals to avoid feeling deprived. Drink water with a slice of lime, or drink soup to feel full. Have a snack if you get hungry for some reason. Avoid eating less than 6 hours before bedtime to prevent insomnia and daytime fatigue. Intermittent Fasting is where someone doesn't eat anything for a set number of hours each day or eats very little and then eats normally again at the end of the fast period. This causes people to lose weight and gain muscle more quickly than usual while also offering many other health benefits.

Even those who are not overweight or obese can benefit from Intermittent Fasting because it is one of the most powerful tools there is for preventing or even reversing diabetes, hypertension (high blood pressure), high cholesterol, and heart disease. It can also reduce the risk of cancer and slow aging. Intermittent Fasting is also an effective treatment for epilepsy, especially in children who are unresponsive to drugs.

Many people don't realize that hundreds of studies have proven that Intermittent Fasting has a wide variety of health benefits. Some have even studied the effects it has on treating cancer, which we will cover in this as well.

So, What is Intermittent Fasting?

Many people don't realize that they are already doing Intermittent Fasting, even if they don't think of themselves as someone who fasts regularly. The truth is that many people eat a very small portion of their daily calories at night and then eat their regular mealtimes during the day. This is intermittent fasting. Another example is people who may only have one meal a day, which means they aren't eating a consistent amount of food every day. However, this person is still consuming nearly all of their daily calories at night and is only eating their normal mealtimes during the day. Intermittent Fasting is simply a more structured way to approach the concepts that many people already do every single day.

Control Your Appetite

Control your appetite and cravings with these tips:

- It's important to stay hydrated while fasting. Drink lots of water and other non-caloric beverages, such as coffee, tea, or artificially sweetened drinks. Avoid alcohol (especially if you're a woman) because it is full of calories.

- Try out new recipes or foods during your fast so that your tastebuds are engaged and ready to go when you break the fast and want to eat some delicious food!

- Sleep a bit longer on your fasting days. This will allow you to have more energy and feel better during the day.

- Track your progress so that you can see all the long-term benefits of Intermittent Fasting. It's also a great way to stay motivated and committed, especially when you are on the last few days of the fast!

- Tell yourself that it is okay if you slip up and eat something while fasting. The goal of fasting is not to feel deprived but rather to create better habits and empower you with information that will help you create a healthier life.

Stick to a Routine

Intermittent Fasting is a type of dieting that cycles between periods of fasting, with either no food or very few foods and periods where you can eat a healthy, balanced diet free from restrictions. Some people find it helpful to plan their fasts so they know when they're going to end and then what they can do in the meantime. The idea is that this makes the fast more achievable in terms of planning for social events and preparing for holidays where there's often temptation around eating more than usual.

This can also be helpful if you're a naturally emotional eater. Fasting when you know it's going to end in a couple of hours can give you something to look forward to. For some people, however, this can be an issue because they see fasting as restrictive, and having rules around it is not helpful.

However, these people find that the more they mentally prepare for fasting and the thought of ending it by looking at an upcoming event or meal as a "reward," the more they feel like planning their fasting regime helps them when their willpower is low. However, it is very important not to overthink it. As you become more used to fasting, the less you'll be thinking about it and the easier it will be, but this does take some time and perseverance.

Give Yourself Time to Adjust

1. **Give yourself time to adjust to an intermittent fasting system.** I've been practicing one for the last 3 months, and it can be a little jarring at first. It gets easier as you get used to it, but there are those moments where you have to remind yourself that this is what sustains you.

2. **Stay hydrated!** Stop drinking fluids at least 2 hours before bedtime because it increases the time needed for food to digest and may disrupt sleep patterns.

3. **Eat nutrient-dense foods!** You want your body to work as efficiently as possible, so getting enough antioxidants, nutrients, and vitamins will help your body function properly during fasts.

4. **Don't starve yourself.** Eat to live!! When I first started fasting, I did not eat enough and starved myself. If you eat too little during the fast, your body will think it is starving and stores fat for survival purposes.

5. **Don't over-exercise!** Exercising too much or at the wrong time can result in dehydration, which breaks down your ability to digest food properly. Also, over-exercising will increase the metabolism, which will also break down your digestion system resulting in weight loss but not fat loss.

6. **Don't over supplement!** Supplementing is not the same as cheating. Cheating your body by taking vitamin and mineral supplements while fasting puts undue stress on your body and causes it to become depleted. This results in weight loss but not fat loss.

7. **Don't mix up phases!!** If you are training hard, try to fast the same amount of time as you would during a training season. If you are continually fasting 90 days a year, then you will have to adjust to 15–18 days of normal eating followed by fasted training cycles.

8. **Don't fast when you are sick.** There is a reason why your body does not digest food when you are sick. My advice is to fast as soon as you feel better.

9. **Don't work out when you are ill or have the flu.** The same advice above! If you have the flu and try to work out hard, it will break down your immune system and make it that much longer for it to operate.

10. **Don't overheat while fasting.** When you overheat, it causes an increase in body temperature, which will also cause your body to not digest properly. This situation could lead to lower energy levels for the rest of the day, or possible illness.

11. **Don't fast if you are pregnant.** I think this one is obvious, but some people will do what they want to do when they want to do it.

12. **Don't eat late at night if you can avoid it.** If you must eat late at night, eat slow-digesting protein and vegetables. A cheeseburger with a bag of chips (starch/sugar) is not going to end well for you!

13. **Get enough sleep!** When we don't get enough sleep, our body goes into panic mode instead of fat-burning mode.

14. **Don't combine Intermittent Fasting with intense exercise.** Listen to your body! If you feel like you're overdoing it, then you probably are.

15. **Don't be in a rush to get fasted!** This is a process, not a race! You want to lose fat and maintain muscle mass, so take your time and enjoy the journey. It will not last forever!

16. **Stay away from things that cause you to stress!** Stress breaks down your immune system causing sickness, which, in turn, results in not being able to train properly, followed by cheating on your eating plan because you do not feel good.

17. **Don't cheat!** Cheating messes with your metabolism, which will cause you to gain weight and not lose fat.

18. **Always do a refeed after fasting.** A refeed is a planned eating event after being on a fast. You need to give your body the fuel it needs for it to function at its best levels. A good time to do a refeed is every 3-4 days, but you can do it sooner if you feel like your body is about to break down because of lack of food intake. A refeed meal is high in protein and carbs!

19. **Get your workout in when you do your refeed.** Give yourself time to digest the food and give your body the energy it needs to get a great workout.

Chapter 11. Differences Between Intermittent Fasting and OMAD (One Meal a Day)

Intermittent Fasting, What Is It, and How Can It Work?

The practices that include abstinence from food have been found in each culture since exceptionally ancient occasions. In fact, fasting can be viewed as an outflow of a serious level of discretion: manifesting itself in the ability that an individual has to control hunger; it addresses the measure of his resolve on one of the most primordial senses of man. This idea has been translated from an alternate point of view and instead went to the impacts on the metabolism and the general state of health: various conventions of food approaches have been examined (and still are) under the name of Intermittent Fasting.

Intermittent Fasting (or intermittent eating regimen) gives several potential applications and sets rules on how meals should be devoured. The research in this regard comes from concentrates on calorie limitation, a nutritional model that accommodates the intake of a lower quantity of calories without any way lessening the stock of fundamental supplements. So, it is about eating less, however better, attempting to enhance our food intake with important supplements.

Initially, the investigations had been carried out on primates: a famous report distributed by a group of American researchers in 2009, in the journal Science, detailed the experience observed on two group of primates, one treated with calorie limitation and the other allowed to eat what they wanted. Twenty years later, the outcomes had been amazing: survival had been significantly higher in the treated group (calorie limitation) than in the untreated group, with a substantial disappearance of constant degenerative diseases like diabetes, heart attack, and tumors.

Later examinations and applications of calorie limitation in humans affirm the old data and are predictable with upgrades in the decrease of disease risks and with the potential anti-aging impacts. The popularity is also because famous individuals use it. In parallel and as of late, conventions have been formulated based instead on Intermittent Fasting or on calorie limitation just inside booked periods, to which alternate times of normal food intake, on a repetitive basis. There are several models:

- 16:8 plan (or also called Leangains) where you fast for 16 hours a day and eat the meals in the remaining 8 hours, generally performed on a maximum of 2 days in seven days.
- Conspire 5:2 (also called "Fast Diet") in which calorie intake imitating fasting is normal (around 500–600 kcal) during 2 days in seven days, while the remaining 5 are eaten normally.
- "Eat-Stop-Eat" plan in which you fast for 24 continuous hours one or 2 days seven days.

- The 16:8 technique is the most well-known and the one that can be applied most easily: it very well may be utilized, for example, by anticipating supper and skipping breakfast the following day.

A week after week timetable may incorporate skipping supper to allow the necessary chance to pass during the evening, taking advantage of the rest phase. Thus, the time window where to eat breakfast and lunch is diminished to 8 hours.

For example, breakfast at 7 am and lunch at 3 pm. In this case, just calories fluids (in this manner without added sugar, yet preferably just water) until 7 am the next morning. As you can see, 16 hours would have passed. You can move the window from 8 to 16 and resume the following morning at 8:00.

It is essential to maintain a certain regularity. Remember that this eating regimen, also called Mima-Fasting, should not to be interrupted by overeating and bad eating. The 16:8 format allows you to join the physical exercise in the afternoon with a sixteen-hour fast.

Different plans, including those not mentioned, then again are hard to follow because of the requirement for exacting planning of both sustenance and sports activities, and I would advise against it, especially for the individuals who are not trailed by a professional (for example, format 18:6 is more complicated, having to wrap two meals in six hours). The outcomes happen if the intermittent eating regimen is protracted over the long haul.

What Is OMAD?

The acronym stands for "One Meal A Day, and it is a kind of system that accommodates the utilization of a solitary meal in the day. This is a solid limit of the idea of Intermittent Fasting since it leads to fasting for 23 hours straight and having a hearty meal in an hour.

Many individuals are adopting this technique for weight control or other health issues, yet there is no uncertainty that, as frequently happens in the food area, it is spreading more as a fashion than for an improvement in one's physical state. In OMAD, the standards are few: the meal should be eaten in the same period of four hours consistently; it is allowing you to consume drinks without calories during the 23-hour fast, and you can eat what you want in the meal for granted.

The positive side is that there is no compelling reason to think about the exact calories or nutritional profile of the food, as long as all the calories are saved for that timeframe; however, the drawbacks are self-evident: not eating for 23 hours will inevitably lead to picking some unacceptable food sources, like high-fat, low-supplement food varieties.

The dangers could be at interrupting the exertion, leading individuals to take in a larger number of calories than necessary, let completely go and pick unhealthy alternatives, as well as the trouble of getting enough supplements that the body needs each day. Also, the exorbitant limitation of this eating routine would lead to a lack of energy, sluggishness, and uncontrollable cravings.

What Are the Advantages of Intermittent Fasting?

Intermittent Fasting is an airtight improvement: it means that if it is dosed in the right way, it creates a reparative and building up the reaction by the body, as happens on account of physical training. This boost is set off by the caloric deficiency and prompts various changes: the body adapts its hormonal levels, the cells initiate the repair through autophagy; also, there is a better insulin reaction.

The impacts of all these changes remember many advantages for health and add to weight reduction, with:

- Improvement of insulin resistance level.
- Decrease in inflammation.
- Changes in the hormonal profile, with an increase in anabolic hormones that advance the mobilization of fats (cortisol, glucagon, testosterone, development hormone.).
- All these consolidated factors bring about a decrease in the danger of creating metabolic diseases, like diabetes, hypertension, cardiovascular disease, and the counteraction of certain kinds of cancer.

Chapter 12. Time-Restricted Feeding

There is more to say about the circumstance of suppers. Sherman and colleagues attempted, consistently on mice, what occurred by giving "garbage" or "sound" eats less, contrasted with giving garbage consumes, fewer calories, yet with a tight food time window (normalizing information as for supplement admission).

Clearly, the mice with the solid eating routine have gotten the best "metabolic incitement" of the sub-atomic pathways of interest with regards to abstaining from excessive food intake, getting thinner, and losing muscle versus fat. Which ones have been more terrible? Those with the eating routine wealthy in low-quality nourishment.

Interestingly, the others have still acquired a decent "metabolic incitement" from the eating routine with lousy nourishment yet with a restricted food window. Citing the specialists: there is a "predominance of 'timed feeding over an eating routine wealthy in fats." Set forth plainly, when you eat is a higher priority than what you eat (on the off chance that we talk about mice for the present).

Any individual who needs to start understanding if things additionally work on people, necessities to check whether they know individuals who eat severely. They will discover that they won't change their food decisions for some time, yet they would already be able to improve their condition by advising them to eat each one of those things (likewise with the same amounts) in a restricted time window.

In any case, let us keep on chipping away at our dear companions with enormous teeth. What occurs on the off chance that you take mice and give them two weight control plans, one sound and one garbage, each furnished with dispersed suppers or with a restricted food window?

- Summing up, in this manner
- Sound eating regimen
- Garbage diet
- Free access (NA)
- Timed admittance (NT)
- Free access (FA)
- Timed admittance (FT)

We could reply by giving a rundown from what gains more weight and deteriorates well-being to what exactly deteriorates less:

FA> FT> NA> NT

Clear and direct: clearly if you do a free garbage diet, you put on weight unreasonably; on the off chance that you do a timed garbage diet, you put on weight; on the off chance that you do a free sound eating routine, you put on a little weight; on the off chance that you do a timed solid eating regimen, you don't put on weight by any stretch of the imagination, to be sure you can get in shape.

Alright, Yet What Amount?

This is the inquiry posed by certain analysts who affirmed the above, yet then saw that the contrast among FT and NA or NT was not very good! The mice ate shoddy nourishment in a timed feeding window, and the impacts resembled what the solid eating regimen gave them. Deciphered: the circumstance "ensured" them from stuffing initiated by the garbage diet. This is the outline diagram (on the off chance that you are thinking "everybody gets fat," in actuality, some portion of the bend is given by the normal expansion in weight because of the development): the defensive impact from swelling of food timing. What's more, here's the delightful contribution from Hatori and colleagues: "a 'time-restricted diet addresses a non-pharmacological procedure against stoutness and related infections."

In short: do you know "nutritionist-safe" individuals, the individuals who simply don't have any desire to proceed to cry at the possibility of somebody driving them to improve their eating routine?

Indeed, simply advise him (model), "Eat what you need; however, do it just between 13 furthermore, 14 and somewhere in the range of 20 and 21." You will, as of now, see enhancements past the conceivable common decrease of what they eat toward the day's end (regardless of whether there were not this, they would, in any case, have upgraded). Time-Restricted Feeding is simply a food "style" in which a fasting period substitutes with a feeding period. This example is the thing that's continued in the Intermittent Fasting.

Would It Be Able to Be Made More Maintainable?

Or on the other hand rather, not every person has the correct inspiration to "not eat" at specific times. There are times when you truly need to plunk down to eat something with family members, companions, associates, or simply chomp on a bite.

Would we be able to, in any case, have the advantages of Timed Restricted Feeding? Would we be able to, in any case, have the ordinary advantages of "delayed" fasting windows (for example, longer than the standard night fast that everybody does)?

The appropriate response is yes. Numerous supporters of Intermittent Fasting believe that only a "complete" fast enables those metabolic pathways; however, it is simply because they have considered the technique (Intermittent Fasting) without understanding the nuts and bolts. You are here to get them, so continue to peruse, and you will realize how to do it. Sugar limitation (or potentially lipid supply) is practically something similar to "Fasting." Since we see that the overall metabolic circumstance is "fast," it doesn't make any difference what is entering upstream because such metabolic and atomic elements at that time are being carried out.

If you give 2,500 calories to a long-distance runner who needs 8,000 calories, it's not quite the same as offering them to the inactive 48 kg young lady. To begin with, those "methods of fasting" will, in all probability, be dynamic. Second, the "methods of anabolism" will presumably be dynamic. In any case, Draznin and associates went a little further and caused us to comprehend that those "fasting pathways" are performed even by overfeeding if this is lipid.

This had effectively been thought about by different investigations (Klein and Wolfe), in which it was clarified, for instance, that managing the "versatile reaction to fasting" isn't the energy limitation, but the starch limitation. Citing Draznin and partners: "Our information demonstrates that an overall decline in carb admission or, albeit less apparently, a general overabundance of fat admission even without a calorie limitation is adequate to initiate the cell energy sensor network AMPK-SIRT-1-PGC1-alpha in human skeletal muscle."

Looking at the situation objectively, narrows the fact that there are a lot of moving towards the decrease of starches and the increment of fats (for example see the Ketogenic Diet) allows a circumstance of this kind: accepted "you eat," yet the body sets up very similar systems which he would do on an empty stomach, just somewhat more insipid.

Fat Fast and Timed CHO Feeding or Lipid Fasting and Timed Glucose Feeding

Fat Fast or Fat Fasting is muddled terms to indicate a fast where you mean to present numerous fats proportionately. Practically speaking, it converts into snacks dependent on lipid sources (nuts, seeds, dim chocolate, coconut). Fasting is "reproduced", as in the very metabolic pathways that would be performed on an empty stomach are implemented, and with comparable benefits (improvement of metabolic adaptability and oxidation of fats, both in the short and medium/long

107

haul). Timed CHO Feeding is a muddled articulation to say Timed Restricted Feeding, where, nonetheless, "fasting" isn't genuine yet recreated, utilizing Fat Fast.

As it was mentioned before, truth be told, starches are by definition restricted (more fat is needed to be added relatively). This implies making not, at this point, genuine fasting time windows substituting with feeding time windows yet exchanging low-carb/high-fat windows (mimicked fasting) with glucose feeding windows. For instance: the first supper of the day hyper lipid/Carbohydrate IPO (or "skipped" on the off chance that you need to do genuine fasting) restricted feeding time window, where starches are additionally embedded.

An adequate illustration of this, destined to show the advantages of overweight individuals from moving starches in the evening, comes from the investigation of Sofer and associates. They have demonstrated that:

1. Straightforward control of sugar conveyance seems to have extra useful impacts when contrasted with an ordinary weight reduction diet in people experiencing stoutness. It can likewise be useful for people experiencing insulin obstruction and metabolic disorder.

2. The weight control plans doled out to the two groups were something very similar; then again, actually, one had sugars conveyed, the other just in the evening dinner. Notwithstanding the extra weight reduction (not all that high), it is most fascinating that there has been a lower transformation to the eating routine

and more prominent food control of the subjects in the test diet (the one with the most sugars in the evening).

3. Before proceeding onward to the real practice, or rather to the utilization of the Intermittent Fasting in a basic manner with the Timed Glucidic Nutrition, we should investigate the advantages of short fasting windows (genuine or mimicked) on different parts of well-being.

Chapter 13. The Solution: Intermittent Fasting

Food Pyramid

Up until this point, the investigations allow us to understand that he metabolic circumstances in which the body is set toward the start of the fasting, is vital for the digestion that will happen through the following stages: "sugar burner" or "fat eliminator". For well-being, weight reduction, and actual wellness, we need "fat consuming food"; eating a more lipid-moving supper or fasting is superior to eating dinners, especially if it is full of carbs.

Food timing can be a higher priority than the amount you eat, as it can ensure weight loss from the impacts incited by the conceivable presentation of garbage, fatty eating routine, or with a blend of high carbs and high fats. With a similar measure of supplements (and calories, on the off chance that you need…) presented, it is smarter to eat fewer dinners regarding weight reduction, metabolic boundaries, and well-being. This is because the living being has a specific upgrade to improve metabolic adaptability by moving it's "fat consuming" digestion because of the presence of fasting stages (genuine or mimicked).

This can allow us to draw up this Intermittent Fasting/Nutrition (starch) food pyramid, where other deciding variables have been added (active work, food mindfulness, booked fasting days). At the base, we track down the timed carbohydrate nutrition. Any dietary methodology should have specific planning of sugars, to abuse the advantages of pretty much little fasting windows (genuine or reproduced). On the second step, we discover the sign on breakfast, either to be skipped or high fat/low carb; on the third step we read, is the thing that we as a whole ought to desire: food mindfulness, underlining the nature of food, at any rate for the greater part of the eating routine. On the fourth step, there is the thing that could we could do 1−2 times each month, or the expansion of the time window to low sugars as long as 72 hours, or a total fast of 24−36 hours (valuable, for instance, after times of "wealth," as after-parties/events/occasions).

We go to the components to dodge or do just "on the off chance that it occurs:" try not to eat simply because the time has come to eat; keep away from inordinate (and outlandish) discontinuity of dinners, predictable carb admission at every feast, starch as it were tidbits and fluid calories—planned carb taking care of the functional setting.

Here is the thing that all of you expected, the application part. In the first place, we present the "skeleton" for setting up a Timed Carbohydrate Feed convention. In the following paragraphs, we present a portion of our models and ideas tested in the field that will cause you to see how effectively you can improve even in "troublesome" cases (for example, when you don't have such a lot of inspiration to begin an organized excursion-which then can generally proceed on the Intermittent Fasting wave!).

In outline, here are the critical ideas to remember for Timed Carbohydrate Nutrition:

1. Enter sugars (carbs) just in a specific time window, not broadened (the sign is 5−6 hours, for example, just 1−2 suppers of the day which can be the lone ones, or be important for a convention with indeed, a few dinners, however of the kind portrayed in point 2).

2. Interference of fasting with moderately hyper lipid, hypoglycaemic, however not very protein feast, (demonstratively 50−60% fat, 10% starches, 40−30% protein), or no interference (which implies that all calories and supplements are amassed in those 5−6 hours); a model could include a few eggs or yogurt with dried products of the soil be finished with small portions of new natural product.

3. Bites—if present—moderately hyper lipid, hypoglycaemic, yet not proteinic, (if they are snacks on the fly, straightforward dried organic product or seeds are great). Here as well, the option isn't to eat anything, everybody will discover their path. Some individuals will understand that they feel better with little dosages of fats and some will feel vastly improved on a total fast.

4. Complete and fulfilling evening dinner (or in the long stretches of more noteworthy unwinding-as we will see in no time): pick all the food classifications (proteins, carbs, fats) and eat, arriving at fulfillment, filling yourself. Getting satisfied doesn't mean "feeling full." However, if you want go further, one way to avoid

eating more could be to stop when you are more parched than hungry; drink 1 glass of water and pause… On the off chance that you are still hungry after 10−20 minutes, you can incorporate another natural product, like yogurt. Otherwise, the dinner closes there.

Plans and Application Models: Insight and Tests

We then present the three conventions we generally use, bare and crude, beginning from the real Timed Glucose Feed. These conventions likewise have names that reflect what comprises of Carbdark: the carb taking care of window is in the evening hours (Timed sugar taking care of appropriate); Pleasure: not indispensable taking care of window, is made (with the suggestion that we will portray) including starches; and Wildabe: feast models made and set by the emotional day (as of now found in Meal Timing for an adaptable eating routine).

Carbdark. Coordinated Carbohydrate Power Supply legitimate This model is the thing that we have called the "diet for supervisors or business visionaries"; it is truly helpful altogether those situations where the responsibilities are set Monday-Friday 8/9: 00−17/18: 00 and there are many collaborating stresses … Essentially, this is valid for 80% of individuals.

Carbdark: how to?

- Fasting
- Taking care of suppositions

- Dinners with max 20-25 g protein, <20 g starches, 15-20 g fat.
- Or, on the other hand, dinners with disconnected fat sources: 15–30 g fat.

Complete blended taking care of:

- 40–60 g protein
- 50–100 g carbs
- 10–30 g fat

Timing:

- 16–18 h
- 6–8 h

Chapter 14. The Best Way to Practice Intermittent Fasting

There are numerous kinds of IF with various alternatives that can adjust to any program or way of life. You have to test and track down the one that works best depending on your necessities. For amateurs, the most straightforward beginning stage is the 16:8 Intermittent Fasting technique, a type of taking care of restricted on schedule. This regularly includes simply avoiding the after-supper nibble and skipping breakfast the following morning as well. On the off chance that you don't eat anything somewhere in the range of 20:00 and 12 the following day, for instance, you have effectively abstained for 16 hours.

Remember that Intermittent Fasting should be viewed as an adjustment in the way of life rather than an eating routine. In contrast to common eating regimens, there is no compelling reason to tally calories or connect food sources in a food journal consistently. To receive the rewards of Intermittent Fasting, make certain to zero in on the nature of your eating routine by picking solid, entire food sources during the days you eat.

Likewise, always tune in to your body. On the off chance that you feel shortcoming or weariness when fasting, attempt a quick bite or tidbit. Then again, you can attempt one of the other Intermittent Fasting techniques and find what works for you.

Intermittent Fasting, the study of taking care of when it comes to nourishment, the emphasis is for the most part on the quality and amount of food: eating as normal food varieties as could be expected and burning through the calories essential for the body without abundance, are two amazing ideas that everybody presently knows to live fit as a fiddle and in well-being. In any case, there is a third factor that is typically not thought about: fleeting supposition. The purported "intermittent fasting" plays exactly on this factor, and lately, it has gotten progressively mainstream, even among athletes.

By definition, Intermittent Fasting is a dietary methodology. It comprises doing diets intermittently, for example, not for a few days ceaselessly but rather just lengthening hours during which you must remain hours without eating, aside from the admission of fluids without calories and dietary benefits.

Natural teas are therefore fine; however, a centrifuged or a concentrate is not because they give the body a progression of substances will turn on the metabolic motor. The objective is rather to kill the digestion of intestinal retention.

Are There Various Application Techniques?

Totally yes. By perusing the web, incidentally, everybody has their say. Intermittent Fasting is a wholesome methodology that operated as an essential strategy in human sustenance, in particular eating the food accessible when it was free. This occurred before the appearance of horticulture and pastoralism, when man lived as an agrarian.

116

What Do You Prescribe to an Individual Who Needs to Attempt This Food Methodology Autonomously?

Initially, a metabolic registration to ensure there are no issues; on the off chance that they exist, you should examine the alternative of assessing Intermittent Fasting with your doctor. Also, I don't prescribe this strategy to a found-out pregnant lady, or a kid, or individuals with specific metabolic illnesses or stories of dietary problems, except if under expert watch.

Except for these cases, the least demanding technique to test Intermittent Fasting is to lengthen the period of the physiological fast that every individual typically encounters during rest, taking out the night fast. This should make possible to skip or postpone breakfast or skipping or expecting supper. These two things should likewise be possible together. Along these lines, the delay extends.

What Are the Base-Long Stretches of Fasting?

At any rate, 14 hours, yet additionally 16 hours.

Along these lines, does the body enter an alternate metabolic state?

Careful. Remember that man has fashioned his hereditary qualities, using a food style that is no longer what it is today. The pattern of three suppers and three tidbits is a custom from about 30 years back.

On remote times, did man eat less?

Indeed, considerably less since he needed to go through his day getting food. He ate once or twice a day, regularly once after food assortment exercises.

Is it safe to say that you are alluding to crude man?

If you take a gander at the most recent agrarian clans, practically every one of them would, in general, eat in the evening as they went through the day searching for food. The disclosure of agribusiness and pastoralism permitted the advancement of human progress as numerous individuals did not need any more to stress over searching for food. Now they could stand to do other exercises not related with the obtainment of food, like craftsmen and smithies.

Is the decision of food free in intermittent fasting?

As indicated by the first culture of man, the right answer is characteristic, sound, and natural eating, whether or not you eat every 3 or 13 hours. This is the presence of mind that I would prescribe to any individual who needs to endure this current negative deviation of human food advancement, food culture. Without going too far back on schedule, our grandparents would not perceive numerous substances on food marks.

What are the remedial and preventive impacts on infections?

There is a lot of logical writing which expresses that intermittent fasting, from a well-being perspective, gives two advantages: metabolic and intellectual well-being. To start with, therefore, it improves metabolic adjustments like weight, diabetes, and related pathologies and afterward psychological ones like feeble dementia and Alzheimer's.

A patient with diabetes should have an assessment from an expert in organizing the right Intermittent Fasting food plan. For this situation, through intermittent fasting, the "match is dominated." In any case, on the off chance that it is at an advanced stage, it is important to assess the metabolic state since, in these cases, the person is not ready to enact certain components and, all things considered, there is no hope. In any case, if Intermittent Fasting is received in the beginning phases of the disease, it is a good methodology.

I give a model: a patient of mine, whose blood glucose values and his family ancestry anticipated an instance of diabetes inside a couple of years. Through a quarter of a year of dietary renovating, he began playing tennis for 2/3 hours per week without issues; at the beginning, he was unable to try and operate from an hour of play.

Yet, it was a beginning phase. In case he had been a high-level diabetic, an insulin dependent; it wouldn't have been conceivable. This likewise applies to Alzheimer's from a psychological perspective; calorie limitation and Intermittent Fasting are equally inadequate in these cases.

For instance, in youthful anorexics, during the underlying stage, before the body starts to self-rip apart (when it burns through muscles to take care of itself), there is a time of expanded psychological capacities where they take great grades at school.

Why do you experience an improvement in intellectual abilities?

This is because a progression of metabolic pathways is activated to improve physical and intellectual performance. With an empty stomach, the lone chance of not biting the dust has the option to get prey, and to do it; you should be more grounded, fast, and cautious. To make a similarity, canines chase after the chase when chasing.

Intermittent Fasting and sports can go inseparably?

In speed and force sports, it is extremely powerful; in high-intensity games, it is important to figure the length of the athletic presentation. Exploration groups have made directed on each kind of population— beginner, and expert athletes—who didn't track down specific oddities. During a fast, it is said, the digestion diminishes.

What occurs in Intermittent Fasting?

The term in these cases is elusive since it fits terrible translations. At the point when the body runs out of supplements and calories, the body responds by entering reserve storage mode. Thus, the facts demonstrate that in outright terms; it goes down; however, it surely doesn't kill or hang, essentially "stairway." Obviously, if an individual doesn't eat, the only way for the body to take care of is to consume its stored saves, and by then, it consumes fat, which is the least difficult thing for the body.

Is there a danger of losing bulk in intermittent fasting?

On the off chance that it is intermittent, there is not, to such an extent, that it is used for the body recomposition of the competitor, such as the individuals who should fall into the weight classes and can't manage the cost of a drop-in execution. Surely, it should be an intermittent fast and not a fast done in the previous three days.

Would you be able to practice for a couple of days?

It tends to be practiced as unpredictably as conceivable since the body adjusts to any propensity.

How is this abnormality "organized?"

In theory, you eat when you feel like it or when it is advantageous, or by receiving various protocols. You can therefore change times, sorts of supplements; sometimes, you can embrace a calorie limitation rather than intermittent fasting. I have two or three books in which I clarify these "sporadic" protocols; inevitably, perusers figure out how to construct one dependent on their experience.

It is therefore significant not to give the body reference focuses.

That is correct because Intermittent Fasting works like intense intermittent pressure; an airtight improvement is characterized. On the off chance that, then again, the pressure is persistent and constant, the talk changes; the body was formed by intense and intermittent pressure. Taking the case of crude man, when a creature pursued him, this was intense pressure because, following a couple of moments, the creature had gone after you or not. In a cutting-edge key, ceaselessly bearing a disagreeable office administrator is an ongoing pressure. The first is a pressure that makes you more grounded; the other debilitates as it crushes the neuro-endocrine-insusceptible framework.

In intermittent fasting, I envision that suppers are all the more full-bodied since similar calories are taken in fewer admissions. Is there a danger of encountering an expansion in glycemic load?

This relies upon the supplements taken in.

Is there a danger of going hungry?

As far as I can tell, I would say no, aside from people with metabolic issues who should be followed up by a trained professional.

Can a competitor train on an empty stomach?

Indeed, except if it is a perseverance movement. On account of short and extraordinary exercises, enduring about 60 minutes, there are no issues.

In this food system, you skip breakfast. However, it is frequently said that it addresses the primary dinner of the day.

No one has at any point stressed where this theory comes from. I think about man's sound judgment and transformative history. In 1600, breakfast was just made by the rich, particularly ladies, since men went chasing; it was a rich game. On the off chance that the man has never eaten, he should not accomplish such a great deal of hurt. I don't think it is manageable to say that morning meal is a key feast, except if bites and bread rolls must be sold.

How would you see starch-rich breakfast cereals?

They are loaded with lousy nourishment. By the way, they are not non-exclusive starches but rather brimming with sugars.

Does Intermittent Fasting additionally decrease food yearnings?

Indeed, since the body creates a progression of neuromodulators that follow up on hunger.

All in all, I envision that humans tune in preferred to actual yearning over a mental craving, that is, the longing for food?

Indeed, as long as you don't begin from a dietary issue, which for this situation establishes one of the prohibition rules.

Is it genuine that with this food technique, you can accomplish more prominent mental fixation, inventiveness, learning, and improved rest quality?

Indeed, except if unreasonable calorie limitations are continued in intermittent fasting, where yearning takes over by then.

Chapter 15. Metabolic Effects of Fasting

As we will see, as per its term, fasting has various repercussions on the living being. A fast of a couple of hours should be thought of; it is to be viewed as physiological; it is true to be told regular, in the existence of any sound individual, not to eat nourishment for a couple of hours (by and large 4 or at least 5 if you don't eat any sort of tidbit) after one of the primary dinners; fasting following typical night's rest is physiological.

Fasting can be recognized by its length. In a most of the cases, we are thinking about four stages: post-assimilation stage, momentary fasting, medium-fasting, long haul fasting. The post-ingestion stage is the one that happens once the food sources that have been taken during dinner have been consumed by the small digestive tract (by chance: the second piece of the small digestive system is classified "fasting"). The stage being referred to has a span of around 4–5 hours, after which, all in all, other food is taken, subsequently interfering with the condition of fasting.

During the post-retention stage, there is, in the typical subject, a drop in blood glucose levels (bringing down of glucose); the body "responds" to this decrease with a cycle known as hepatic glycogenolysis (debasement of glycogen particles until glucose is shaped), important both for keeping up sufficient glycemic levels and for providing glucose with different tissues of the body.

125

In momentary fasting, quantifiable in one day of abstention from food, the metabolic requirements of the body are upheld, notwithstanding liver glycogenolysis, additionally by the oxidation of fatty oils; the glycogen contained in the liver, indeed, is somewhat restricted and it is accordingly important for the body to turn to unsaturated fats to save glucose (proposed principally for the brain and red platelets).

The living being then uses a metabolic interaction known as gluconeogenesis; through this cycle, glucose is blended utilizing non-glycidyl antecedents (amino acids, glycerol, lactic corrosive, pyruvate, and so on). Gluconeogenesis (likewise neo glycol beginning) has the basic role of adding to the consistent support of the blood glucose fixation.

Following 24 hours of fasting, you pass into the medium-fasting stage; during this stage, there is a somewhat checked emphasis on the advancement of the gluconeogenesis interaction. The amino acids that are abused for this cycle are those getting from the debasement of the proteins contained in the muscle tissues (in the organic human entity, there are no stores of proteins usable for energy purposes); indeed, we are seeing what is to some degree characterized as "cannibalization of the muscles" with ensuing diminishing in bulk. The presence of indications like shortcomings, weariness, and indifference are unavoidable.

The gluconeogenesis cycle tends, over the long run, to lose viability, to such an extent that the inventory of glucose to the mind is small; in this manner, the utilization of ketone bodies (CH3)2CO, vinegar acetic acid derivation, and 3-B-hydroxybutyrate gets fundamental; these get from lipid digestion; truth be told, without sugars, lipids can't be used for energy purposes, and the living being is compelled to change them into ketone bodies, substances that have certain qualities that make them like sugars, as a matter of first importance their astounding information speed and speed of utilization.

Ketosis has the beneficial outcome of extending the endurance of human beings. However, the "results" are not definitive. Simply notice the impressive expansion in blood acridity and work load to which two significant organs, for example, kidneys and liver, are exposed to discard the body's overabundance of ketones. As fasting perseveres, the different tissues, to save however much glucose as could reasonably be expected, are constantly compelled to resort progressively to lipid oxidation.

After the twenty-fourth day of fasting, the last period of fasting is passed; without mediation, the subject is bound to bite the dust inside a perceptibly short time. The organic entity, indeed, has abused every one of the assets that the liver and blood made accessible to him, and the passing comes due to breathing troubles, drying out, and breakdown of the safe framework. As a reference, an individual can make due about a month of fasting, even though instances of longer diets have been recorded.

Helpful (Discontinuous) Fasting

Taking into account what is accounted for in the past passages, it is feasible to make a few contemplations on the topic of helpful fasting, that is, of that fasting which, utilized for periods and with suitable

127

frequencies (hence it is additionally called discontinuous), can improve our well-being. On the off chance that, previously, fasting was essentially connected to enchanted strict decisions, today it is seen fundamentally as a type of actual sanitization, disposal of poisons that should have dirtied our body following an off-base eating routine.

Despite the way that often the individuals who talk about fasting can embed a noteworthy arrangement of logical cautionary while clarifying the supposed advantages of the activity, it is feasible to show how fasting, even incidental, is unsafe. Truth be told, during a calorie decrease, humans can do a transformation or convenience measure.

With the variation, there is a bringing down of the basal digestion to protecting the assets, while with the convenience, the assets are utilized to make up for the absence of supplement supply. By and large, the creature will, in general, use transformation measures that are not dangerous (for instance, the fit body isn't influenced). With fasting, almost certainly, settling cycles will happen, particularly if it is extended.

Indeed, gluconeogenesis (for example, the utilization of lipids and proteins to get the glucose important to keep up ordinary blood glucose esteems; in a stationary, glycogen stores are depleted in under 24 hours) effectively following a couple of days produce negative effects: the lean mass is influenced to change over proteins into energy (with ensuing liver over-burden) and fats (with a thinning impact) with the resulting collection of ketone squander are additionally utilized for a similar reason. Restorative fasting, as opposed to decontaminating the life form, inebriates it!

Restorative Fasting

Contingent upon its length, fasting has various repercussions on humans. Also, fast one day? One day fasting is additionally not positive. Indeed, a stationary (for a competitor, it is difficult to quickly and train) who has a calorie prerequisite of 1,800–1,900 calories spends around 1,400 of them for the basal metabolic rate. This implies that to live, the living being, if fasting, produces waste. Decontamination doesn't rely upon fasting, however, but on the capacity to dispense with these squanders; if this capacity comes up short or essentially diminishes, fasting can't reestablish it.

Thus, one should ask when fasting begins to hurt, mindful that great won't ever do. The appropriate response is in the slag sum, which the gluconeogenesis interaction produces by dismantling the muscles and consuming fat within sight of low or amazingly low sugar stores to have important energy.

Since gluconeogenesis is utilized to compensate for an absence of energy, the harm to fasting relies upon the energy spent by the subject: it is one thing to fast while lying in bed, and the other is to fast while carrying on with a functioning life. Indeed, even a day's fast can hurt.

A tale: a kid abstained for around 36 hours because of a gentle influenza disorder that had influenced the gastrointestinal lot. Having to recoup,

129

operated from his disease, he thought it well to play a debilitating ball game.

Result: tear to the adductors. There could be no counter-test; however, almost certainly, the protein catabolism set off by fasting, and actual exertion caused the injury.

Fasting as Indicated by Elective Medication

As indicated by some hygienist flows, fasting would likewise have a remedial capacity (as we have seen, they call it helpful fasting) and even would mend numerous illnesses, including tumors, on account of a cycle of cell autolysis that would cause tissue reestablishment.

This hypothesis is just an illustration of how obliviousness of the bases of human physiology will, in general, help inventive, simply philosophical speculations, totally disconnected from the real world. Unnecessary to remark, I can just refer to the instance of a partner of mine who, after having accepted elective hypotheses, veganism, and others as such for quite a long time, was struck at a little more than 50 years old by a tumor in his digestive tract (a sickness that can be dealt with today with opportune traditional intercession); he rejected all therapy and, until the end, accepted that fasting could save him. Honor to consistency, yet maybe the kids and spouse would have favored that he was as yet alive.

Imagining that fasting can decontaminate is common to anorexic attitudes who anyway accept that food or a few food sources can do a great deal of damage. It's a given fact that in a solid individual, it isn't clear why slag should accumulate (Which? Where? In what amount?), which would be wiped out by fasting. Given that it is fasting that inebriates the body; if an individual isn't in offset with his eating regimen (that is, he can't normally cut the waste it produces), it implies that he eats in a disorganized way.

Chapter 16. Myths About Fasting

Many myths are related to fasting. These myths have been rehashed frequently to such an extent that they are regularly seen as obvious certainties.

Part of these myths are:

1. Fasting places you in hunger mode.
2. Fasting resembles starving.
3. Fasting causes indulging when eating once more.
4. Fasting makes you lose bulk.
5. Fasting denies the group of supplements.
6. Fasting causes hypoglycemia.
7. The mind needs glucose to work.
8. It is hard to do.

Since quite a while ago denied; however, these myths endure. If they were valid, none of us would be alive today. Think about the outcomes of muscle loss since energy creation. In the long winters, there have been numerous days when our predecessors had no food. After the first experience, they would have genuinely debilitated. After a few rehashed scenes, they would have been powerless to the point that they couldn't chase or gather food. Man, as an animal category, could have never endured.

There is another diligent legend that synapses need glucose to work appropriately. This isn't correct. The human brain, novel among creatures, can use ketones as the principal fuel source during a delayed craving, allowing the preservation of skeletal muscle proteins. Once more, the results of glucose should be considered significant for endurance. Man, as an animal type, would not endure; following 24 hours, the glucose runs out, and we would become nitwits when our brain breakdowns. Our mind, our lone benefit over wild creatures, starts to vanish. Individuals would vanish soon. Fat is how the body stores long-haul food energy, and glucose/glycogen is the momentary arrangement. At the point when momentary energy stores run out, the body effectively goes to long-haul energy stores. Accordingly, on account of the body, glucose is utilized for momentary energy and fat for long haul energy stockpiling. Fat isn't burned if there is a ton of glucose accessible. The bountiful glucose accessible over many years prompts an expansion in fat stores.

What Might Occur if Glucose Was Not, at this Point, Accessible? Would All that Mood Killer in "Hunger Mode?"

No, the energy that is put away with as much consideration as fat would be delivered. The method of appetite, as it is famously known, is the strange "individual of color" who has consistently been appeared to startle us and not make us miss even a supper. Inside a year, about 1000 dinners are devoured. Over 60 years, this compares to more than 60,000 suppers.

To believe that skirting 3 suppers would do hopeless harm to the 60,000 that have been devoured is crazy. Lysis of muscle tissue happens at incredibly low muscle to fat ratio levels or roughly 4%. Thus, it's hardly anything a great many people need to stress over. If we had resulted in these present circumstances point, it would imply that there is no more muscle to fat ratio to activate for energy, and accordingly, slender tissue is assembled.

The human body has advanced to endure wordy times of appetite. Fat is stored energy, and muscle is practical tissue. Fat is burned first. For what reason would it be a good idea for us to expect that the human body is so inept? The body keeps up bulk until muscle versus fat turns out to be low to such an extent that it must choose between limited options.

Thusly, fasting isn't suggested in a BMI of under 19 or within sight of genuine constant illnesses with natural decay. Investigations on intermittent fasting, for instance, show that worry about muscle loss is generally strange. The variation of day-by-day fasting for 70 days diminished body weight by 6%, yet fat mass diminished by 11.4%. Slender mass (counting muscle and bone) has not changed by any stretch of the imagination. Critical enhancements in LDL cholesterol and fatty substance levels have been noticed, and also a developing of chemical increments to keep up bulk. Investigations of burning fat through an intermittent fasting routine have discovered more noteworthy fat loss, regardless of a similar calorie admission. Significantly, no proof of muscle loss has been found.

The other constant legend of the "hunger methodology" is that the basal metabolic rate is altogether diminished, and our body digestion is "killed." This is additionally extremely hurtful for the endurance of the human species. If our digestion goes down after only one day of fasting, we would have less energy to chase or gather food. With less energy, we are less inclined to get food. With every additional day, we are considerably more vulnerable, which makes us even less inclined to get food.

This is an endless loop whereby the human species would not have to endure. It is ludicrous! Indeed, there are no creatures or human species intended to eat three dinners every day. We have effectively seen in different investigations that the basal metabolic rate increments during fasting; it doesn't diminish. The digestion is sped up; it doesn't go out.

It isn't clear where this fantasy comes from. The day-by-day calorie limitation (common to ordinary eating regimens) prompts a decrease in basal metabolic rate, so the analysts estimated that this would deteriorate during fasting as food consumption dropped to nothing. It isn't so. If we rely upon food admission for energy, the decline in food prompts a decrease in energy, which is related to less energy use. Nonetheless, if the food admission goes to nothing, the body passes the energy consumption from the food we eat to the stored food or the fat of our body. Every one of the unbelievable advantages of fasting doesn't occur on a low-calorie diet.

Truth be told, just 7.5 grams of glucose (2 teaspoons of sugar or a taste of soda pop) is sufficient to switch ketosis. Very quickly after burning through glucose, beta-hydroxybutyrate and acetoacetate ketones drop to just about nothing, as do unsaturated fats. Insulin increments, as does glucose.

What's the Significance Here?

The body quits consuming fat. Presently we should return to consuming the sugar we eat. There are rehashed fears that fasting can prompt gorging. Calorie consumption concentrates after a fasting period shows a slight increment at the following feast. Following a one-day fast, the normal calorie consumption increments from 2436 to 2914; yet for the entire 2-day time frame, there is still a net shortage of 1958 calories. The expansion in calories scarcely compensated for the fasting day calorie shortfall. If you are worried about micronutrients and minerals, you can generally take multivitamin planning. Another routine, like rotating intermittent fasting, can likewise alleviate worry about supplement lack.

Science is clear. Myths about fasting are simply lies. There are various fasting regimens. There just is no "greater" type of fast. They are largely useful for various individuals, in various degrees. Similarly, as some favor chicken hamburger steak, there is nobody right or wrong answer. A routine works for one individual; however, it very well may be inadequate for another. Fasting is characterized as the willful demonstration of swearing off nourishment for a specific timeframe. Non-calorie beverages, for example, water and tea, are permitted. Total fasting alludes to swearing off food and drink. This should be possible for strict purposes. For example, during Ramadan in the Muslim practice, however, it is not suggested for well-being purposes, as a result of the lack of hydration it causes.

Fasting doesn't have a standard term. The fasting period can differ from twelve hours to a quarter of a year or more. You can take a fast once every week, once a month, or once per year. Intermittent fasting includes standard fasting for more limited periods. More limited fasting periods are normally more continuous. The longest fasting periods are generally 24 to 36 hours, a few times each week. Shorter fasting can last from seven days to a month.

Conclusion

If you've been reading the Internet for a while, you may have heard of Intermittent Fasting. You might have been looking for diet tips or how to lose weight quickly. So, what makes Intermittent Fasting different from the usual calorie restriction and exercise? Intermittent Fasting (IF) is a method of eating where you restrict your food intake on certain days, then eat normally on others. The process has medical benefits far beyond just weight loss, with notable studies showing that it can lower cholesterol levels and blood pressure, improve insulin sensitivity, and even make aging brains more resilient against Alzheimer's-type damage.

But the biggest benefit of Intermittent Fasting for women might be that it can reduce your risk of heart disease. This is the conclusion of a new study by researchers from Johns Hopkins and Harvard Medical School. The scientists found that women who ate only four days a week increased their lifespan by 3.1 years, lowered their blood pressure, and improved their lipid profiles. Their fasting days were Thursdays, Fridays, and Saturdays. Fasting also helped women lose a bit of weight because they consumed fewer calories. But it's not the only way to lose weight in this manner; you don't have to fast four days a week if you can't squeeze it into your busy schedule.

How Does Intermittent Fasting Work?

The researchers who conducted the study showed promising results for both human trials and animal studies when fasting for only one day per week. Because of these results, the scientists decided to test their theory on female mice and human subjects. Both groups of women participated in an eight-week study. Fasting days were either Wednesday, Friday, or Saturday, and they ate only during the other three days of the week. During two weeks before starting the intermittent fasting, all the women consumed an unrestricted diet. Then at the start of each two weeks, without any messaging or instructions given before, they were asked to adjust their eating patterns so they would eat every day except for fasting days. When the trial ended, the results showed that the women benefited greatly from fasting just one day a week, even though their daily calorie intake remained higher than during their unrestricted diet.

The Benefits of Intermittent Fasting for Women

The researchers found that short-term fasting reduced blood pressure in humans, and a previous study had determined that fasting can reduce elevated cholesterol levels. According to Dr. Richard Isaacson, director of the Alzheimer's Prevention Clinic at New York-Presbyterian/Weill Cornell Medical Center, "Fasting may be an alternative mechanism to protect against neurodegeneration." Another study found that people who fasted once a month had less cognitive decline than those who did not fast at all.

Intermittent Fasting is a bit more complicated than you might expect, but the benefits and health perks far outweigh any minor inconveniences. The longer you can put off food, the more weight you'll lose. Just remember to always eat a healthy breakfast and drink plenty of water the day after you fast.

Fasting significantly improves cholesterol profiles by reducing an enzyme that converts cholesterol to fatty acids, giving it instead of a place in your cell membrane (which prevents heart disease). Also, research shows that fasting can boost stem cells in your body and perhaps play a role in maintaining healthier brain cells. Additionally, Intermittent Fasting has many other benefits like improving cardiovascular health, heart rhythm regulation and helps some with diabetes manage their condition better.

The best part about Intermittent Fasting is you can do it anytime, anywhere, without any restrictions. You don't have to go on a strict regimen or sacrifice your social life. Intermittent Fasting has become a popular lifestyle choice, which is why many dietary institutions are studying the possibility of creating programs for their members.

If you haven't tried Intermittent Fasting before, here's an example: On Monday and Tuesday, fast for 16 hours like normal, then eat all the food you want on Wednesday and Thursday (according to your appetite), as long as it does not exceed 20% of your caloric goals. The same goes for Saturday and Sunday, when you can eat whatever amount of calories is necessary to meet your caloric goals for that day.

Intermittent Fasting is when you choose an eating window (most people choose 8 hours), and for the other 16 hours of the day, you abstain from any food or drink. This doesn't mean that if it's 9 am at this moment, then at 10 am, your body will require nourishment—it means that between midnight and 8 pm (or whatever your chosen time frame is), nothing goes into your mouth on those days.

Some people do this every day, but that's not necessary. It's called Intermittent Fasting because you fast intermittently. Some days you'll choose to fast for 18 hours, and the next day you'll fast for 20 hours. Some people might even choose to go a full 36 hours without food— that's up to you and your body. There are many ways to break up your eating window. 8 hours is the most popular because it fits in perfectly with workday schedules, but some choose a 14-hour window or even just 10, 12, or 15 hours as well. It depends on personal preference and schedule with work/life/etc.

Low-Carb Diets are a type of Intermittent Fasting because you skip breakfast, lunch, or both. People who do this style of fast often eat dinner and then don't eat again until lunch the next day. That is also known as the 5:2 diet, which is popular in the U.K. and has been talked about in news outlets such as The Guardian. It's named that because you normally eat for 5 days a week and restrict calories to 500 per day for 2 days each week. This is just one way to do Intermittent Fasting, but it's becoming more popular due to how effective it can be at weight loss, overall health, and eating less processed foods during your eating window. Keep in mind that you should consult your doctor before starting a fasting regimen.

Lightning Source UK Ltd.
Milton Keynes UK
UKHW020628060521
383207UK00003B/278